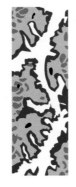

ATLAS OF BONE MARROW AND BLOOD PATHOLOGY

ATLASES IN
DIAGNOSTIC SURGICAL PATHOLOGY

Consulting Editor
Gerald M. Bordin, M.D.
Department of Pathology
Scripps Clinic and Research Foundation

Published:

Wold, McLeod, Sim, and Unni:
Atlas of Orthopedic Pathology

Colby, Lombard, Yousem, and Kitaichi:
Atlas of Pulmonary Surgical Pathology

Wenig:
Atlas of Head and Neck Pathology

Kanel and Korula:
Atlas of Liver Pathology

Owen and Kelly:
Atlas of Gastrointestinal Pathology

Virmani, Burke, and Farb:
Atlas of Cardiovascular Pathology

Ro, Grignon, Amin, and Ayala:
Atlas of Surgical Pathology of the Male Reproductive Tract

Wenig, Heffess, and Adair:
Atlas of Endocrine Pathology

Ferry and Harris:
Atlas of Lymphoid Hyperplasia and Lymphoma

Kern, Silva, Laszik, Bane, Nadasdy, and Pitha:
Atlas of Renal Pathology

Clement and Young:
Atlas of Gynecologic Surgical Pathology

Forthcoming Titles:

Brooks:
Atlas of Soft Tissue Pathology

Silverberg:
Atlas of Breast Pathology

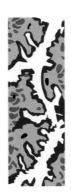

ATLAS OF BONE MARROW AND BLOOD PATHOLOGY

Faramarz Naeim, M.D.
Professor of Pathology and Chief of Hematopathology
UCLA Department of Pathology and Laboratory Medicine
UCLA Medical Center
Los Angeles, California

W.B. SAUNDERS COMPANY
A Harcourt Health Sciences Company
Philadelphia ■ London ■ New York ■ St. Louis ■ Sydney ■ Toronto

W.B. SAUNDERS COMPANY
A Harcourt Health Sciences Company

The Curtis Center
Independence Square West
Philadelphia, Pennsylvania 19106

Library of Congress Cataloging-in-Publication Data

Naeim, Faramarz.
Atlas of Bone Marrow and Blood Pathology / Faramarz Naeim.—1st ed.

p. ; cm.

ISBN 0–7216–8735–0

1. Bone marrow—Diseases—Atlases. 2. Blood—Diseases—Atlases. I. Title.
[DNLM: 1. Hematologic Diseases—pathology—Atlases. 2. Bone
Marrow—pathology—Atlases. WH 17 N143a 2001]

RC645.7.P377 2001

616.4′1—dc21   00-032234

ATLAS OF BONE MARROW AND BLOOD PATHOLOGY   ISBN 0–7216–8735–0
Copyright © 2001 by W.B. Saunders Company.

Printed in the United States of America.

Last digit is the print number: 9   8   7   6   5   4   3   2   1

To

Ester, Shiva, Arash, and Behnaz

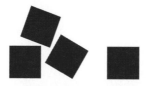

PREFACE

The main purpose of this atlas is to provide easy and quick access to information and guidelines on bone marrow and blood pathology to practicing physicians and those in pathology or hematology training. The text and images are designed to improve diagnostic and classification skills of the reader by a multidisciplinary approach, with primary emphasis on morphology. Histologic and cytologic findings are correlated with relevant ancillary tests, such as special cytochemical stains, immunophenotypic features, and cytogenetic and molecular studies.

The first two chapters provide basic information regarding normal hematopoiesis and a general overview of abnormal bone marrow morphology. Chapters 3 through 10 are devoted to premalignant and malignant conditions. Disorders representing monolineage involvement of monocytic/histiocytic, granulocytic, lymphocytic, erythroid, and mega-karyocytic series are discussed in Chapters 11 through 15. Chapter 16 is devoted to bone marrow hypoplasia, and Chapter 17 offers a brief presentation of bone marrow transplantation. The general format of discussion, for most disease categories, includes pathologic features, clinical aspects, and differential diagnosis.

FARAMARZ NAEIM, M.D.

ACKNOWLEDGMENTS

I am grateful to Carol Appleton for her assistance in the development of the images. I greatly appreciate the contributions of Diana Tanaka-Mukai and Cecille Repinski in the selection of cases with interesting blood, bone marrow, and flow cytometric findings. I would also like to thank Dr. Sunita Bhuta, Department of Pathology and Laboratory Medicine, UCLA School of Medicine, for her contribution of electron microscopic figures, and Dr. Nagesh Rao, Department of Pathology and Laboratory Medicine, UCLA School of Medicine, for his contribution of cytogenetic images. I am grateful to the residents, fellows, and my other colleagues for their assistance and their constructive remarks.

FARAMARZ NAEIM, M.D.

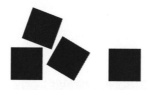

CONTENTS

CHAPTER 1

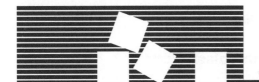

Normal Bone Marrow Structure and Blood Cells

Bone marrow is a mesenchymal-derived complex structure consisting of hematopoietic precursors and a heterogeneous supporting microenvironment. All hematopoietic cells including lymphocytes, erythrocytes, granulocytes, macrophages, and platelets are derived from multipotent bone marrow stem cells (Figure 1–1).

Stem cells have highly specific homing properties, demonstrate very high self-renewal potential, and are capable of differentiation. They share morphologic features of blast cells and are distinguished by their functional properties and expression of certain differentiation-associated macromolecules. For example, multipotent stem cells express CD34, but do not express CD38 and HLA-DR, whereas CD34$^+$, CD38$^+$, and/or HLA-DR$^+$ progenitor cells represent committed stem cells.

Bone marrow microenvironment is composed of stromal cells, vascular structures, a complex extracellular matrix, and regulatory cytokines that are produced by a variety of hematopoietic and stromal cells (see Figure 1–1). The regulatory processes in hematopoiesis are based on place-dependent, cell-cell, cell-matrix, and cell-substrate (cytokine) interactions that link genetic activities to the events affecting the cell surface in coordinated processes.

The self-renewal and differentiation of the progenitor cells in the bone marrow result in daily production of billions of mature cells that are released into the circulation. Therefore, normal bone marrow consists of a heterogeneous population of cells in various stages of differentiation and maturation, while normal blood contains only end-stage and close to the end-stage mature cells.

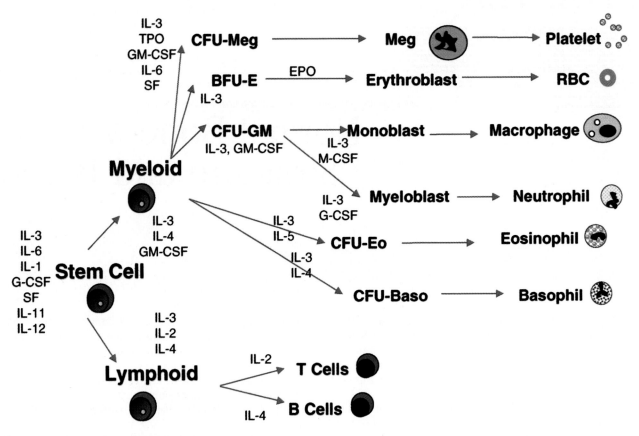

Figure 1–1. Current scheme of hematopoiesis demonstrating the differentiation of the multipotent stem cell to hematopoietic precursors and mature blood cells and showing various levels of cytokine interaction.

BONE MARROW EXAMINATION

Bone Marrow Sections

Bone marrow sections are used for the estimation of bone marrow cellularity and for the identification of structural abnormalities and pathologic processes, such as granulomatosis, amyloidosis, fibrosis, metastasis, and hematologic malignancies. Bone marrow cellularity is defined as the percentage of the bone marrow occupied by hematopoietic cells (% cellularity = bone marrow area minus area occupied by fat). Cellularity of the bone marrow depends on the location of the marrow sample and age of the individual. It is usually higher in the vertebrae and lower in the ribs than in the iliac crest. Bone marrow cellularity approaches 100% at birth, and declines approximately 10% for each decade of life. Thus, in a 50-year-old healthy person, bone marrow cellularity is about 50% (Figure 1–2).

Bone marrow sections are routinely stained with hematoxylin and eosin (H & E) and sometimes with Giemsa stains. They are of two types: biopsy sections and marrow particle sections (Figures 1–3 and 1–4). Marrow particle sections are prepared from aspirated bone marrow, and thus, they represent only cell types and lesions that are released by aspiration. In this book, all the demonstrated figures of the bone marrow sections represent H & E stain unless otherwise specified.

Bone Marrow Smears

Smears are prepared from the marrow aspirates and are usually stained with Wright's and/or Giemsa stains (see Figures 1–3 and 1–4). They are used primarily for the study of maturation steps, cellular details, differential counts, and assessment of the myeloid:erythroid (M:E) ratio (normal range = 2–3). They are also useful for cytochemical stains and evaluation of the bone marrow iron store. In this book, all the demonstrated figures of the bone marrow and blood smears represent Wright's stain unless otherwise specified.

Bone Marrow Touch Preparations

Touch preparations (imprint smears) are made by gently touching (pressing) the glass slides over the biopsy sample and are usually stained with Wright's and/or Giemsa stains (see Figure 1–3). They often show significant artifacts, but are the only source of cytologic evaluation when bone marrow aspiration fails to yield marrow (dry tap). In this book, all the demonstrated figures of the bone marrow touch preparations represent Wright's stain unless otherwise specified.

Bone Marrow Cells

Granulocytic Series

Granulocytic series include neutrophilic, eosinophilic, and basophilic/mast cell lineages. The morphologic steps in the maturation process of the granulocytic series include myeloblast, promyelocyte, metamyelocyte, band cell, and segmented cell (Figures 1–5 and 1–6). During this process, the nuclear:cytoplasmic ratio decreases, cytoplasm accumulates lysosomal granules that are nonspecific at first (primary granules, azurophilic granules) and become specific (secondary granules) later, the nuclear chromatin becomes coarser and denser, and the nucleoli appear less prominent and indistinct.

Myeloblasts are characterized by a high nuclear:cytoplasmic ratio, a centrally located round or oval nucleus, finely dispersed chromatin, and several nucleoli. They are divided into three types based on their cytoplasmic granularity: type I, containing no cytoplasmic granules; type II, containing less than 20 cytoplasmic azurophilic granules; and type III, containing more than 20 cytoplasmic azurophilic granules (see Figure 1–5).

Promyelocytes have more cytoplasm and larger quantities of azurophilic granules than myeloblasts. They show a perinuclear pale area (a well-developed Golgi system) and an eccentric round or oval nucleus. Because type III myeloblasts and promyelocytes share overlapping morphologic features, their distinction at times is difficult (see Figure 1–5). Myeloblasts are HLA-DR+ and may express CD34, whereas promyelocytes are negative for HLA-DR and CD34.

Myelocytes and *metamyelocytes* are intermediate cells characterized by abundant cytoplasm, predominance of specific granules, coarser chromatin, and lack of distinct nucleoli (see Figure 1–6). *Band cells* and *segmented cells* are the end-stage cells and are characterized by nuclear lobulation. Neutrophilic bands (stabs) are cells with bilobed nucleus with no filaments, and neutrophilic segmented cells (segs) demonstrate up to five distinct nuclear lobules (segments) connected to each other by filaments (Figure 1–7).

Eosinophils and basophils undergo more or less similar differentiation steps. Mature *eosinophils*, unlike segs, usually have bilobed nuclei and are loaded with eosinophilic granules. Eosinophilic granules are larger than the neutrophilic granules (Figure 1–8). Mature *basophils* contain a large number of coarse basophilic granules and show less nuclear segmentation than the neutrophils (see Figure 1–8). *Mast cells* are closely related to the basophils and are characterized by abundant cytoplasm packed with ba-

sophilic granules and a round or oval nucleus (see Figure 1–8).

Monocyte/Macrophage Lineage

Monocytes and macrophages are derived from the same committed stem cells (colony-forming unit–granulocyte macrophage, CFU-GM) as the granulocytic cells. The maturation process in this lineage starts from *monoblast*, and then goes through *promonocyte, monocyte, macrophage (histiocyte)*, and *multinucleated giant cell* (such as osteoclasts or giant cells in granulomas) (see Figures 1–5 and 1–7). Monocytes are released from the bone marrow into the blood, and then they migrate out of the circulation into the various tissues and finally transform into different types of macrophages or tissue histiocytes, such as soft tissue histiocytes, pulmonary alveolar macrophages, and hepatic Kupffer cells.

Iron is stored in bone marrow macrophages as hemosiderin (insoluble aggregates) or less abundantly as ferritin (soluble). Prussian blue (potassium ferrocyanide) stains hemosiderin as dark blue cytoplasmic granules (Figure 1–9).

Erythroid Precursors

The morphologic steps in the maturation process of the erythroid series include erythroblast (rubriblast, pronormoblast), prorubricyte (basophilic normoblast), rubricyte (polychromatophilic normoblast), and metarubricyte (orthochromic normoblast) (Figure 1–10). During this process, the nuclear:cytoplasmic ratio decreases, cytoplasm accumulates hemoglobin, the nuclear chromatin becomes denser and pyknotic, and the nucleoli appear less prominent and indistinct. Metarubricyte eventually extrudes its nucleus and becomes reticulocyte (polychromatophilic red blood cell). Reticulocytes gradually lose their ribosomes (in 1–2 days) and become mature red blood cells (RBCs).

Platelet Precursors

The earliest morphologically identifiable platelet precursor is megakaryoblast (promegakaryoblast, group 1 megakaryocyte) (Figure 1–11). Megakaryoblasts undergo endomitosis (nuclear division without cytoplasmic division) once or twice and become promegakaryocytes (group II megakaryocytes). Endomitosis continues and the cell volume gradually increases, and the end result is the formation of granular megakaryocytes (group III megakaryocytes), which are able to release platelets (see Figure 1–11). Megakaryocytes are the largest hematopoietic cells in the bone marrow.

Lymphoid Lineage

Lymphocytes, similar to the other hematopoietic cells, are derived from the multipotent stem cells. Lymphoblasts, the earliest morphologically identifiable lymphoid cells, have a high nuclear:cytoplasmic ratio with a narrow rim of dark blue nongranular cytoplasm, a round or oval nucleus with fine chromatin, and one to two nucleoli. Mature lymphocytes are slightly larger than erythrocytes, and are characterized by scanty blue cytoplasm, round nucleus, coarse chromatin, and inconspicuous nucleolus (see Figure 1–7). The lymphoid maturation results in the formation of two major groups of cells: T lymphocytes and B lymphocytes. A small proportion of lymphocytes, both in the bone marrow and blood, are large lymphocytes with abundant cytoplasm and cytoplasmic azurophilic granules. These *large granular lymphocytes* (LGL) are more frequently identified in normal blood smears than

bone marrow smears (Figure 1–12). They are of two types: Natural killer (NK) cells (CD3⁻ and CD8⁺) and cytotoxic T cells (CD3⁺ and CD8⁺). LGL cells often express CD16, CD56, and/or CD57 molecules.

Hematogones are bone marrow B-cell precursors that are $CD10^+$, $CD19^+$, $HLA-DR^+$, and TdT^+, and may express CD34. These cells may morphologically resemble lymphoblasts, but usually show somewhat denser chromatin and absent or inconspicuous nucleoli (see Figure 1–12).

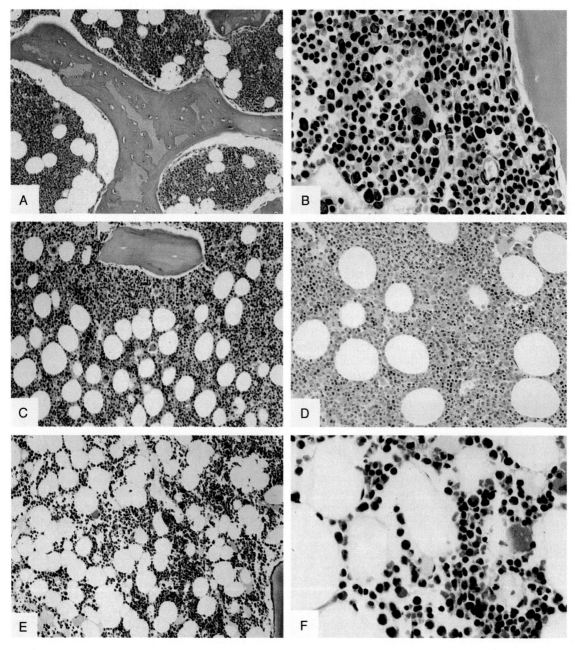

Figure 1–2. Bone marrow cellularity declines by age. Biopsy sections from 2-year-old (*A* and *B*), 55-year-old (*C* and *D*), and 75-year-old (*E* and *F*) individuals.

Prolymphocytes are larger than lymphocytes (more cytoplasm and a larger nucleus), display a coarse chromatin and often show a prominent nucleolus. They are either of B- or T-cell origin (see Figure 1–12).

Activated lymphocytes (transformed B or T cells) are large cells with abundant cytoplasm and a highly polymorphic nuclear morphology (see Figure 1–12). They are more frequently identified in blood smears than in marrow smears.

Plasma cells are the end product of the B-cell lineage and are characterized by abundant dark blue cytoplasm, a pale perinuclear area (Golgi system), and an eccentric nucleus with coarse chromatin (cartwheel appearance) (Figure 1–13).

Lymphoid aggregates are relatively common findings in bone marrow sections, particularly in the elderly. They are well-defined structures primarily consisting of small mature lymphocytes (see Figure 1–13).

Other Bone Marrow Cells

Other bone marrow cells include osteoblasts, osteoclasts, adipocytes (lipocytes, fat cells), fibroblast-like cells, and endothelial cells (Figure 1–14).

Text continued on page 12

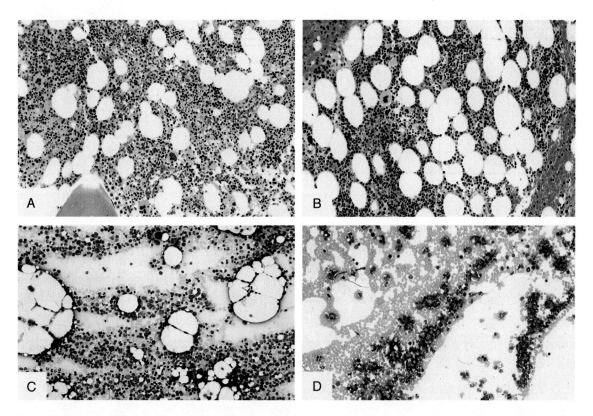

Figure 1–3. Bone marrow sample preparations. Biopsy section *(A)*, clot section *(B)*, aspirate smear *(C)*, and touch preparation *(D)*.

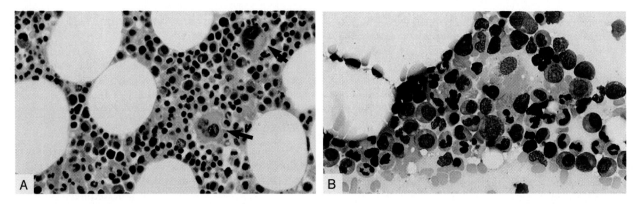

Figure 1–4. Bone marrow clot section *(A)* and marrow smear *(B)* demonstrating a mixture of erythroid and myeloid precursors at various stages of maturation. Megakaryocytes are several times larger than the other bone marrow cells, have abundant cytoplasm, and show a large, highly lobulated nucleus *(A, arrows)*.

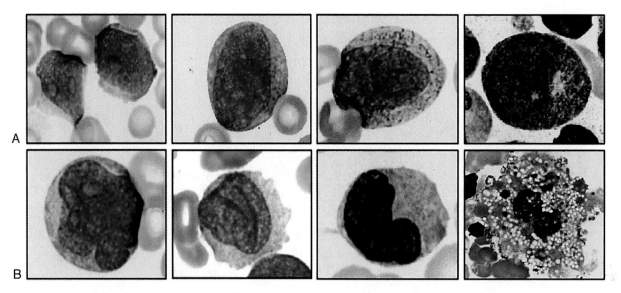

Figure 1–5. Left to right: *A* demonstrates types I, II, and III myeloblasts and a promyelocyte; and *B* shows monocytic maturation from monoblast to promonocyte, monocyte, and macrophage.

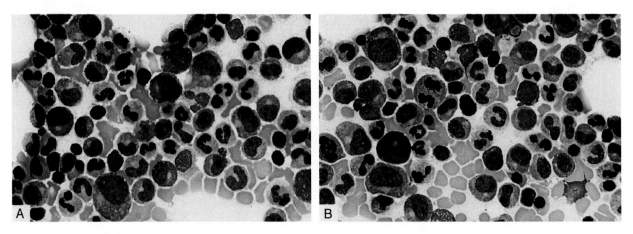

Figure 1–6. Bone marrow smears *(A* and *B)* demonstrating myeloid cells in various stages of maturation.

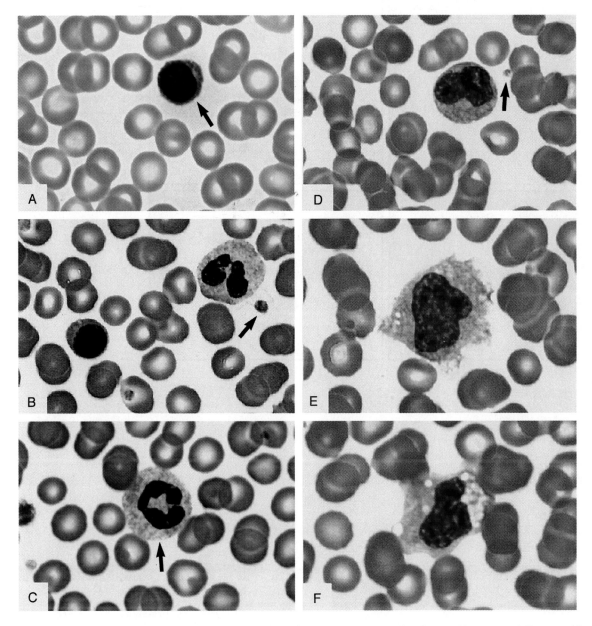

Figure 1–7. Blood smears demonstrating normochromic, normocytic erythrocytes *(A–F)*, mature lymphocytes (*A, arrow,* and *B*), neutrophils (*B* and *C, arrows*), platelets (*B* and *D, arrows*) and monocytes in various shapes and sizes, some with cytoplasmic vacuoles *(D–F)*.

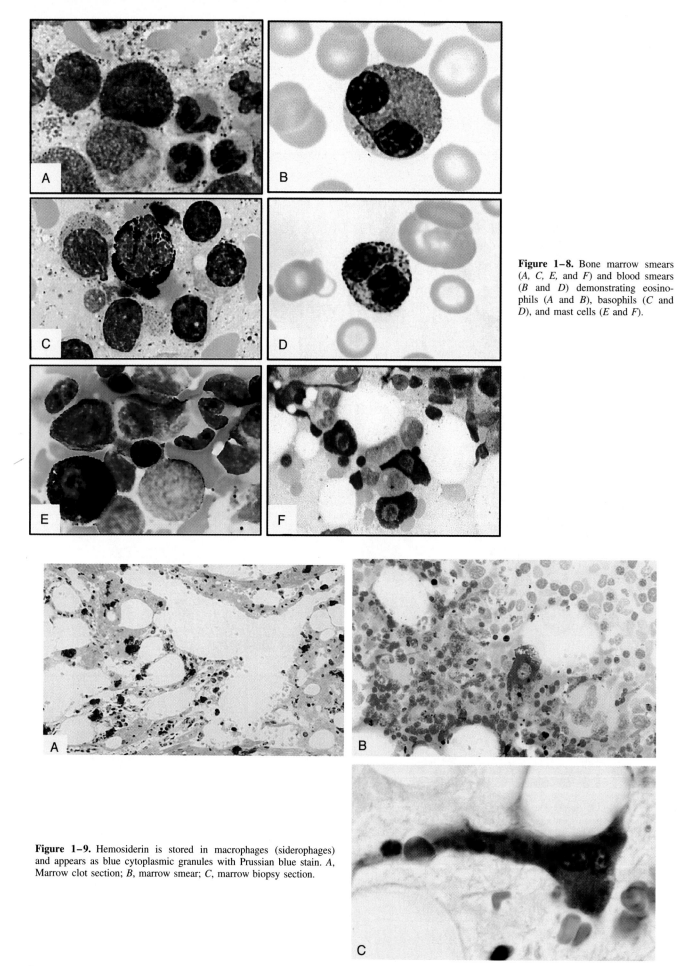

Figure 1–8. Bone marrow smears (*A, C, E,* and *F*) and blood smears (*B* and *D*) demonstrating eosinophils (*A* and *B*), basophils (*C* and *D*), and mast cells (*E* and *F*).

Figure 1–9. Hemosiderin is stored in macrophages (siderophages) and appears as blue cytoplasmic granules with Prussian blue stain. *A,* Marrow clot section; *B,* marrow smear; *C,* marrow biopsy section.

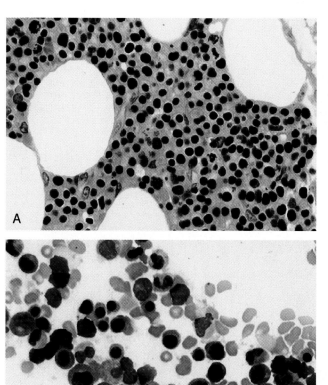

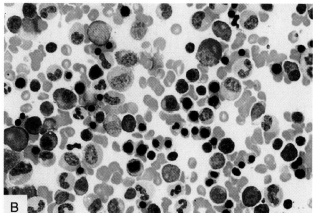

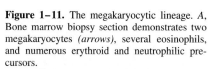

Figure 1–10. Erythroid and myeloid precursors at various stages of maturation. *A*, Bone marrow biopsy section; *B* and *C*, bone marrow smears.

Figure 1–11. The megakaryocytic lineage. *A*, Bone marrow biopsy section demonstrates two megakaryocytes *(arrows)*, several eosinophils, and numerous erythroid and neutrophilic precursors.

Illustration continued on following page

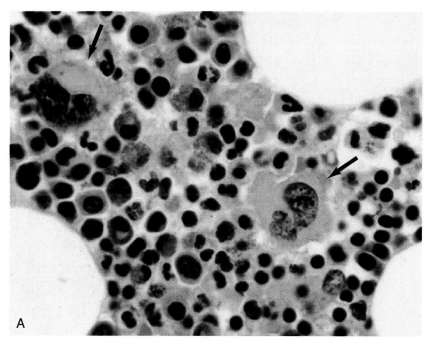

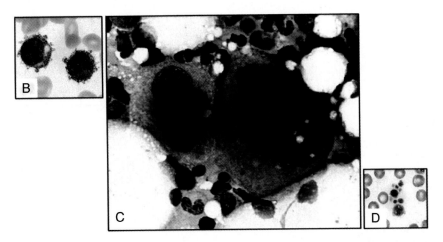

Figure 1–11 *Continued. B,* Bone marrow smear shows megakaryoblasts with cytoplasmic budding; *C,* Bone marrow smear demonstrates megakaryocytes; *D,* Blood smear shows a cluster of platelets.

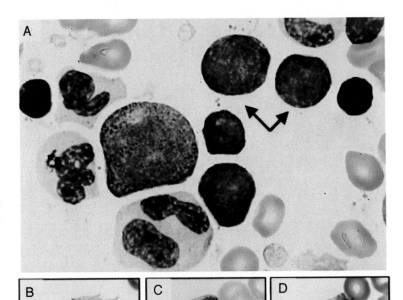

Figure 1–12. The lymphoid lineage. *A,* Bone marrow smear demonstrating B-cell precursors, hematogones *(arrows); B, C,* and *D* are blood smears showing a large granular lymphocyte, a prolymphocyte, and an activated lymphocyte, respectively.

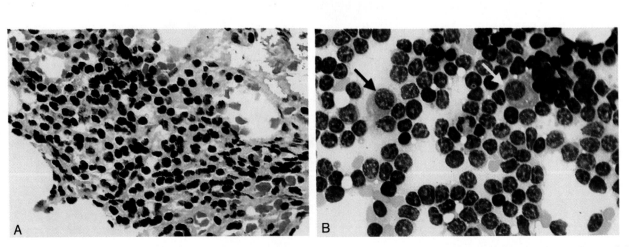

Figure 1–13. A lymphoid aggregate demonstrated in bone marrow biopsy section *(A)* and in marrow smear *(B).* Two plasma cells are also noted *(B, arrows).*

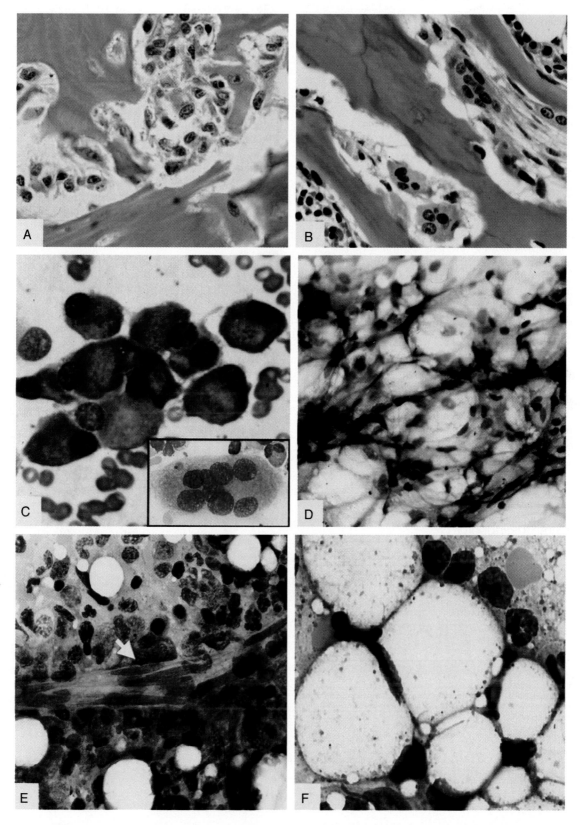

Figure 1–14. Osteoblasts, osteoclasts, adipocytes, and endothelial cells. *A* and *B*, Bone marrow biopsy sections demonstrating osteoblasts and osteoclasts, respectively. *C*, Bone marrow smears showing a cluster of osteoblasts with abundant blue cytoplasm, eccentric nucleus, and perinuclear pale area. A multinucleated osteoclast is shown in the inset. *D*, Bone marrow smear consisting of stromal cells and fatty tissue. *E*, Bone marrow smear showing elongated endothelial cells *(arrow)* surrounded by hematopoietic cells. *F*, Bone marrow smear demonstrating adipocytes.

BLOOD SMEAR EXAMINATION

Blood smears should be thin, evenly distributed over the glass slides, and quickly air-dried and stained (Wright's stain is the most popular stain). Evaluation of a blood smear is a good practice in a routine hematology work-up. A normal complete blood count (CBC) may not necessarily mean normal hematopoiesis. For example, in hereditary spherocytosis, lead poisoning, or malaria, the CBC may be within normal limits, but the peripheral blood smears show spherocytes, basophilic stippling, or RBC-containing parasites, respectively.

Red Blood Cell Morphology

In normal conditions, RBCs are relatively uniform in shape and size, normocytic (an average of 7–8 μm in diameter), normochromic (the pale central area less than 1/2 of the RBC diameter), and contain no inclusions (see Figure 1–7). One to two percent of erythrocytes are larger and polychromatophilic (bluish-red) (Figure 1–15). These represent reticulocytes (see Figure 1–15). Except in newborns, nucleated red cells are not normally found in peripheral blood.

Leukocyte Morphology

The mature leukocytes present in the peripheral blood in normal conditions are neutrophilic segmented cells (segs) and bands (stabs), lymphocytes, monocytes, eosinophils, and basophils (see Figures 1–7 and 1–8). The white

blood cell (WBC) count range is 3 to 10 $\times$ 10^3 cells/μL, with a differential count as shown in Table 1–1.

Platelet Morphology

Platelets are the end products of the megakaryocytic lineage and are released into circulation as cytoplasmic fragments of granular megakaryocytes. They are the smallest hematopoietic elements (measuring 2–4 μm in diameter), with a count ranging from 150,000 to 400,000/μL (see Figures 1–7 and 1–11). A rough estimate of the platelet count is calculated in wedge smear preparations by the number of platelets per oil-immersion field $\times$ 20,000. Approximately 7 to 21 platelets are found per 100$\times$ oil-immersion field in an evenly distributed normal blood smear. Anticoagulants or agglutinins (IgM or IgG), which are found in patients with autoimmune disorders, chronic liver disease, or malignancy, may cause platelet aggregation.

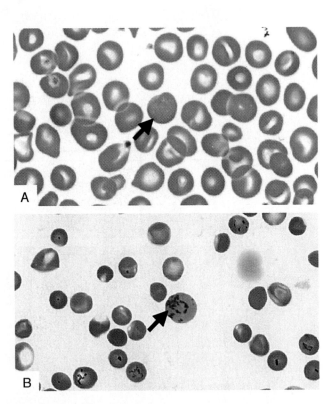

Figure 1–15. Blood smears demonstrating a polychromatophilic erythrocyte *(A, arrow),* and reticulocytes *(B, arrow,* methylene blue stain).

Table 1–1
LEUKOCYTE MORPHOLOGY

Type*	Range (%)
Granulocytes	
Segs	33–72
Bands	0–13
Eosinophils	0–6
Basophils	0–3
Lymphocytes	16–48
Monocytes	1–13

*Certain conditions such as exercise, emotional disturbances, menstruation, anesthesia, convulsive seizures, and electric shock may be associated with a transient neutrophilic granulocytosis. This is due to the demargination of the neutrophilic granulocytes. The presence of immature leukocytes in the peripheral blood should be considered abnormal.

BONE MARROW AND BLOOD EVALUATION CHECKLISTS

The following lists are provided as guidelines for the evaluation and interpretation of bone marrow samples and blood smears:

Bone Marrow Section and Smear:

Estimate bone marrow cellularity.

Look for focal or diffuse lesions (e.g., granuloma, fibrosis, metastasis).

Perform differential count and estimate M:E ratio.

Check megakaryocytes (adequate, reduced, increased).

Check abnormal morphology.

Check presence of iron stain.

Review blood smears or have access to the CBC and differential count.

Have access to clinical information and other laboratory findings.

Blood Smear:

Check RBC morphology (e.g., anisocytosis, poikilocytosis, target cells).

Estimate polychromatophilic RBCs (reticulocytes).

Look for rouleaux formation.

Check WBC morphology and differential count.

Search for immature leukocytes.

Look for RBC or WBC inclusions.

Estimate the platelet count and check platelet morphology.

Selected References

Carr J, Rodak B: Clinical Hematology Atlas. Philadelphia, WB Saunders, 1999.

De Bruyn PPH: Structural substrates of bone marrow function. Semin Hematol 18:179, 1981.

Foucar K: Bone Marrow Pathology. Chicago, ASCP Press, 1994.

Gulati GL, Ashton JK, Hyun BH: Structure and function of the bone marrow and hematopoiesis. Hematol Oncol Clin North Am 2:495, 1988.

Naeim F: Topobiology in hematopoiesis. Hematol Pathol 9:107, 1995.

Naeim F, Moatamed F, Sahimi M: Morphogenesis of the bone marrow: Fractal structures and diffusion-limited growth. Blood 87:5027, 1996.

Naeim F: Pathology of Bone Marrow. Baltimore, Williams & Wilkins, 1997, p 1.

Tavassoli M, Yoffey JM: Bone Marrow Structure and Function. New York, Alan R. Liss, 1983.

Ziegler BL, Kanz L: Expansion of stem and progenitor cells. Curr Opin Hematol 5:434, 1998.

CHAPTER 2

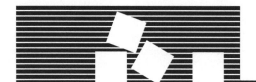

Abnormal Morphology

STRUCTURAL ALTERATIONS

Structural alterations of bone marrow are demonstrated best on tissue sections. The changes include abnormal cellularity, fibrosis, necrosis, gelatinous transformation, metastasis, granulomas, amyloidosis, and vascular and bone abnormalities.

Abnormal Bone Marrow Cellularity

A variety of pathologic conditions are associated with bone marrow hypercellularity (Figure 2–1). Myelodysplastic syndromes, myeloproliferative disorders, and leukemias often display a hypercellular marrow. Conditions that require bone marrow response and overproduction to compensate for cell loss (hemolytic anemia, hemorrhage) or to accommodate increased cellular needs (infections, high altitudes) are also associated with bone marrow hypercellularity. Metastatic lesions may occupy a high proportion of the involved bone marrow and be highly cellular.

Acquired aplastic anemia, Fanconi's anemia, and paroxysmal nocturnal hemoglobinuria (PNH) are associated with bone marrow hypocellularity (see Figure 2–1). Bone marrow samples obtained shortly after chemotherapy, irradiation, or bone marrow transplantation also are hypocellular.

In patients who receive cancer chemotherapy, in posttransplant patients, and in elderly individuals, the cellular distribution of the bone marrow is usually uneven with densely cellular foci between markedly hypocellular areas.

Bone Marrow Fibrosis

Bone marrow fibrosis is a relatively common phenomenon seen in association with a wide variety of pathologic conditions. Fibrosis may appear as a diffuse process such as in hairy cell leukemia and primary myelofibrosis (Figure 2–2), or may be focal or patchy, such as in metastatic neoplasms, chronic renal disease, granulomas, and Paget's disease (Figure 2–3). Reticulin and trichrome stains are useful for the detection of bone marrow fibrosis.

Bone Marrow Necrosis

The most frequent conditions associated with bone marrow necrosis are hematologic malignances and metastatic tumors. The primary cause of marrow necrosis is ischemia. Ischemia may result from vascular occlusion (sickle cell anemia, fibrin clot, tumor emboli, or tumor compression) or inadequate blood supply (circulatory failure, severe anemia, starvation, or fast tumor growth). Chemotherapy and certain infections, such as mucormycosis, Q fever, typhoid fever, tuberculosis, and histoplasmosis, have been associated with bone marrow necrosis. Bone marrow sections show coagulation or fibrinoid necrosis, and bone marrow smears contain amorphous cell debris and pyknotic nuclei (Figure 2–4).

Amyloidosis

Amyloid is an eosinophilic, amorphous, hyaline extracellular deposit. It has been associated with primary (idiopathic) systemic amyloidosis, chronic inflammatory diseases, and monoclonal gammopathies. Amyloid deposits are usually found within the walls of small vessels or adjacent stromal tissues (Figure 2–5). Congo red and methyl violet stains are routinely used for the detection of amyloid deposits. Under polarizing microscope, Congo red stain depicts amyloid as apple-green birefringent deposits.

Granulomas

Bone marrow sections, particularly biopsy specimens, are the best resources for the detection of granulomas. Granulomas are collections of epithelioid histiocytes often surrounded by lymphocytes and plasma cells (Figures 2–6 to 2–9). The most prominent causes of granulomas are sarcoidosis and mycobacterial and fungal infections. However, other infectious and noninfectious conditions, such as syphilis, viral infections, typhoid fever, Q fever, malignant lymphomas, and drug-induced and autoimmune-related inflammatory responses, may develop bone marrow granulomas. Granulomas may contain multinucleated giant cells and/or areas of necrosis. Certain bone marrow lesions, such as metastatic renal cell carcinomas, large cell lymphomas, and mast cell aggregates, may resemble granulomas.

Gelatinous Transformation

Accumulation of hyaluronic acid (gelatinous material) in bone marrow is often associated with fat atrophy and bone marrow hypoplasia (Figures 2–10 and 2–11). This condition, referred to as gelatinous transformation, has been associated with a variety of chronic debilitating disorders, particularly anorexia nervosa. Gelatinous transformation may be mistaken for necrosis, amyloidosis, or edema. The amorphous glassy or finely granular gelatinous material reacts positively with alcian blue and periodic acid-Schiff (PAS) stains.

Acquired Immunodeficiency Syndrome

Bone marrow examination in patients with acquired immunodeficiency syndrome (AIDS) frequently demonstrates various degrees of dysplastic hematopoiesis, eosinophilia, and plasmacytosis (Figure 2–12). Focal or diffuse reticulin fibrosis, gelatinous transformation of bone marrow, or evidence of hemophagocytosis may be present. Patients treated with azidothymidine (AZT) may show megaloblastic changes (see Figure 2–12) or bone marrow hypoplasia. An immune-associated thrombocytopenia with increased marrow megakaryocytes has been observed in some of the patients with AIDS. Bone marrow may also show evidence of lymphomatous involvement or opportunistic infections.

Metastasis

Metastatic lesions usually appear as clusters of atypical cells, larger than hematopoietic cells (Figures 2–13 to 2–17). They are often associated with variable degrees of fibrosis and may show areas of necrosis. The extent of the bone marrow involvement ranges from minimal focal infiltration (micrometastasis) to virtually complete replacement of the bone marrow. In bone marrow smears, metastatic tumor cells are found as well-defined clusters, usually at the periphery of the marrow particles. Metastatic lesions may sometimes simulate marrow fibrosis, osteosclerosis, granulomas or primary hematologic disorders. Additional sections and/or immunohistochemical stains may help to detect these lesions, particularly micrometastases.

Post-Therapeutic Changes

Morphologic features of the bone marrow after chemotherapy and/or irradiation are marked hypocellularity, edema and dilatation of sinuses, necrosis, mild to moderate increase in reticulin fibers, and increased number of macrophages (Figure 2–18).

Bone marrow often shows significant changes following growth factor/interleukin therapy, such as treatment with granulocyte colony-stimulating factor (G-CSF), granulocyte-macrophage colony-stimulating factor (GM-CSF), or interleukin 3 (IL-3). The changes include increased cellularity, dysplastic changes, myeloid left shift, and sometimes eosinophilia. IL-3 may be associated with marrow fibrosis and G-CSF may cause marked dysplasia and myeloid left shift simulating myelodysplastic syndrome or even acute myelogenous leukemia (Figure 2–19).

Bone Changes

Osteopenia is associated with thin bone trabeculae and expansion of the bone marrow space. On the other hand, osteosclerosis is demonstrated by increased thickness of bone trabeculae. Biopsy specimens obtained from previous biopsy sites may show features of chronic inflammation and repair evidenced by new vascularization and proliferation of fibroblasts, edema, increased number of macrophages, and new bone formation (Figure 2–20).

Text continued on page 25

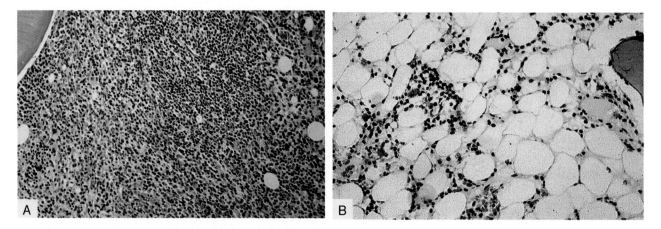

Figure 2–1. Abnormal bone marrow cellularity. Biopsy sections from a 70-year-old male patient with myelodysplastic syndrome *(A)* and a 25-year-old female patient with aplastic anemia *(B)* demonstrate hypercellular and hypocellular bone marrows, respectively.

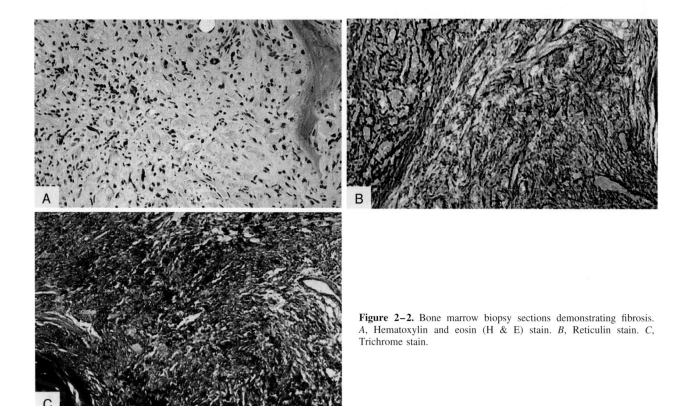

Figure 2–2. Bone marrow biopsy sections demonstrating fibrosis. *A*, Hematoxylin and eosin (H & E) stain. *B*, Reticulin stain. *C*, Trichrome stain.

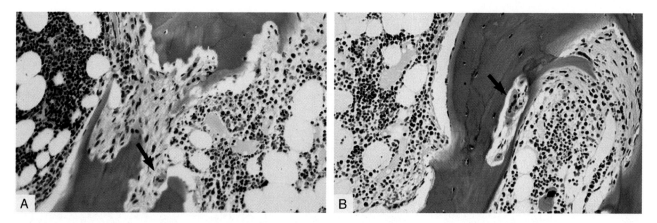

Figure 2–3. Bone marrow biopsy section from a patient with chronic renal failure demonstrating paratrabecular fibrosis, bone remodeling, and the presence of osteoclasts *(arrows)*.

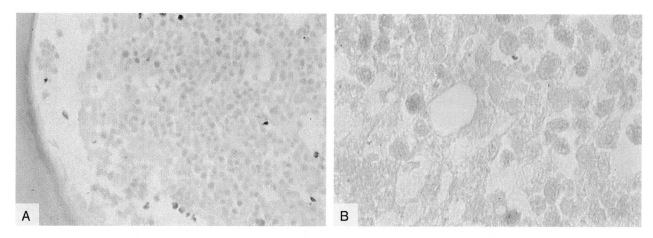

Figure 2–4. Low- *(A)* and high-power *(B)* views of a bone marrow biopsy section showing coagulation necrosis. The shadow of the necrotic cells is visible.

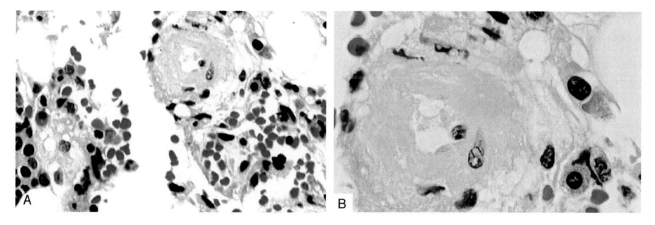

Figure 2–5. Low- *(A)* and high-power *(B)* views of a bone marrow biopsy section demonstrating vascular wall thickening and hyalinization secondary to amyloidosis.

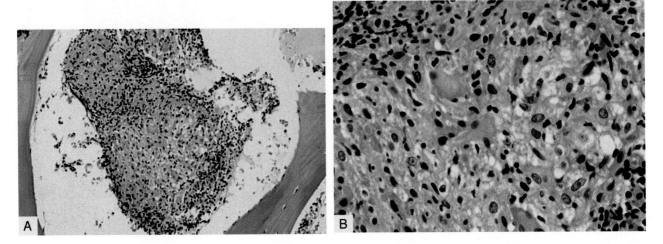

Figure 2–6. Low- *(A)* and high-power *(B)* views of a bone marrow biopsy section showing nonnecrotizing granulomas caused by sarcoidosis.

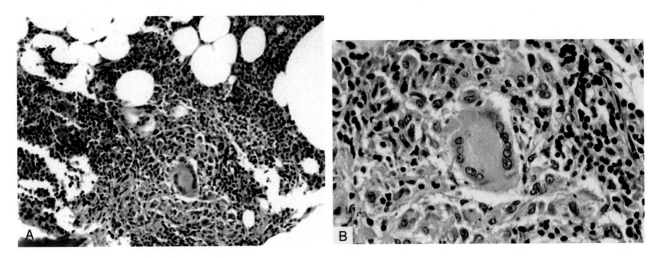

Figure 2–7. Low- *(A)* and high-power *(B)* views of a bone marrow biopsy section from a patient with sarcoidosis demonstrating nonnecrotizing granuloma with a multinucleated giant cell.

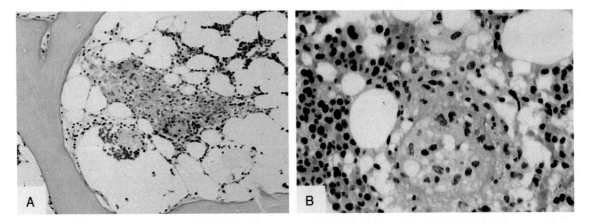

Figure 2–8. Small granulomas composed of epithelioid histiocytes *(A–D)*. Granulomas are often surrounded by lymphocytes and plasma cells *(A–C)*.

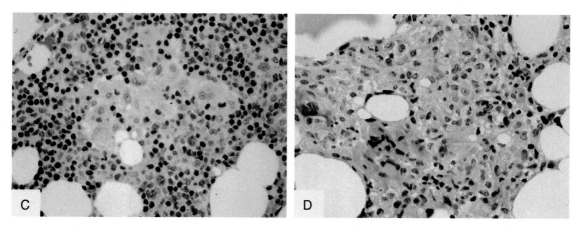

Figure 2–8 *Continued*

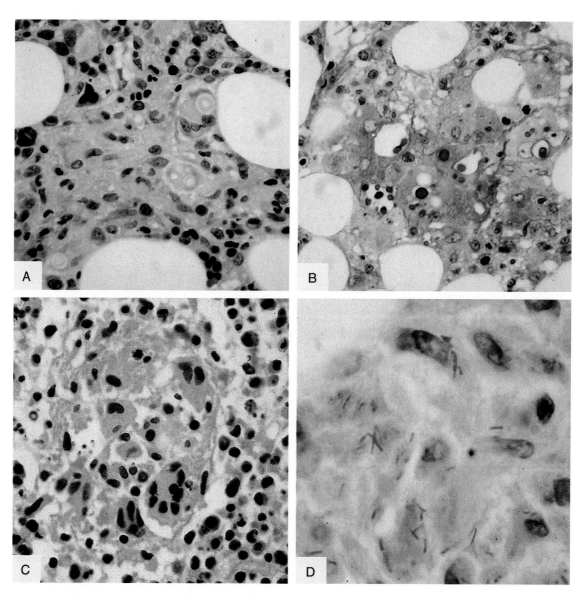

Figure 2–9. The epithelioid histiocytes in granulomas may contain microorganisms such as *Cryptococcus neoformans* demonstrated by the H & E stain *(A)* and periodic acid-Schiff (PAS) preparation *(B)* or *Mycobacterium avium-intercellulare* depicted by an acid-fast stain *(D)* in a bone marrow granuloma *(C)* from a patient with acquired immunodeficiency syndrome (AIDS).

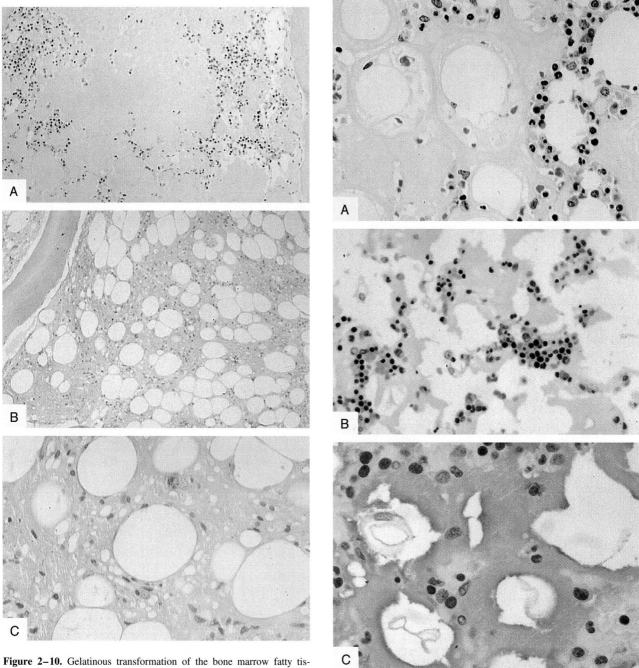

Figure 2–10. Gelatinous transformation of the bone marrow fatty tissue. Biopsy sections are hypocellular, and the bone marrow fat is partially or diffusely replaced by a homogenous eosinophilic substance *(A)*. The substance stains light blue with alcian blue stain *(B* and *C,* low- and high-power views).

Figure 2–11. Gelatinous transformation of the bone marrow fatty tissue. Biopsy sections are hypocellular and the bone marrow fat is partially or diffusely replaced by a homogenous eosinophilic substance *(A)*. The substance appears reddish-pink with PAS stain *(B)* and blue with alcian blue stain *(C)*.

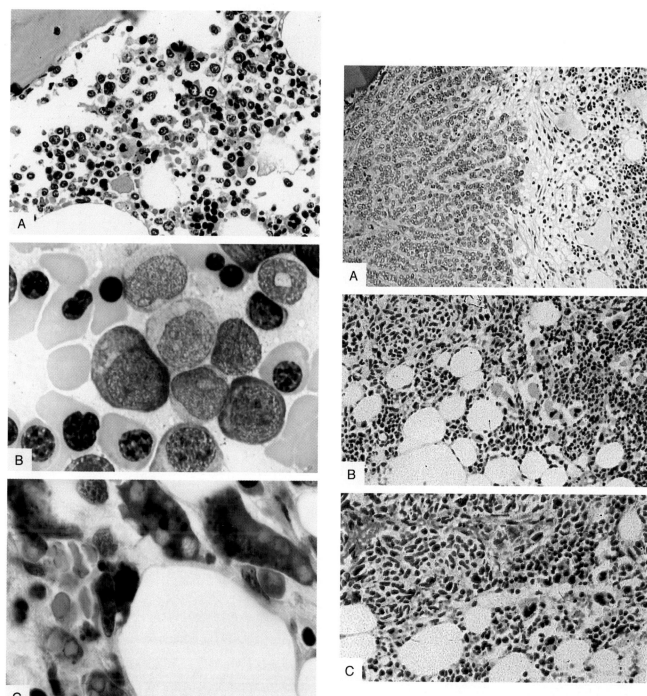

Figure 2–12. Bone marrow biopsy section *(A)* from a patient with AIDS demonstrates hypercellularity and plasmacytosis. Bone marrow smear *(B)* shows megaloblastic and dysplastic changes. Bone marrow biopsy section stained with a combination of H & E and Prussian blue stains *(C)* depicts iron-loaded macrophages with evidence of hemophagocytosis.

Figure 2–13. Bone marrow metastasis. Metastatic neoplasms may appear as well-defined focal lesions separated from hematopoietic cells by a fibrous band *(A)* or may show no stromal reaction and mix with the hematopoietic cells *(B and C).*

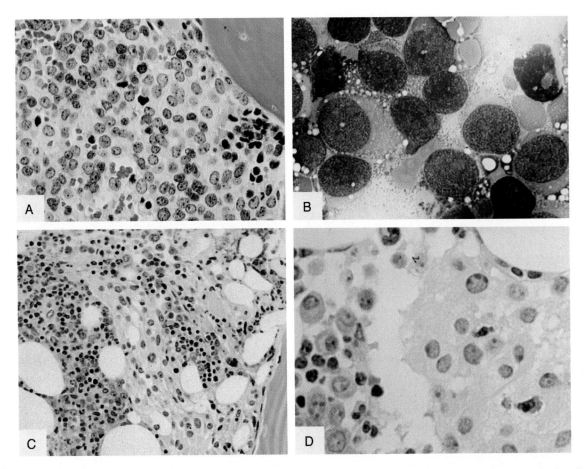

Figure 2–14. An example of metastatic rhabdomyosarcoma is demonstrated in *A* (biopsy section) and *B* (marrow smears). The neoplastic cells appear as round primitive cells with frequent mitotic figures *(A)*. An example of metastatic pheochromocytoma is presented in *C* and *D* (biopsy section, low- and high-power views). The tumor cells show minimal nuclear pleomorphism and have abundant clear cytoplasm.

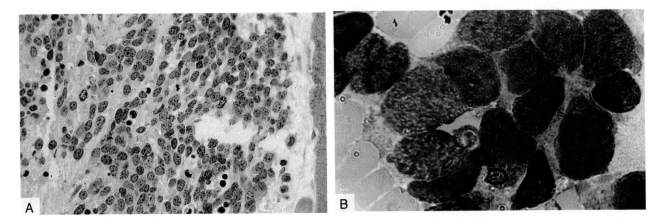

Figure 2–15. An example of metastatic neuroblastoma is demonstrated in *A* (biopsy section) and *B* (marrow smear). The neoplastic cells appear as round primitive cells with frequent mitotic figures *(A)*. Special stains for neuron-specific enolase, synaptophysin, and chromogranin all were positive (results not shown).

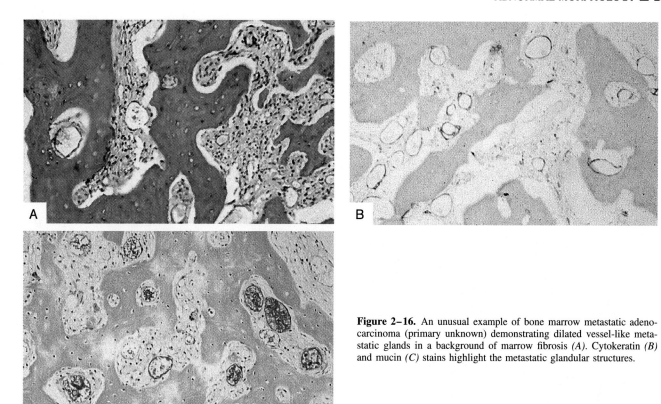

Figure 2–16. An unusual example of bone marrow metastatic adenocarcinoma (primary unknown) demonstrating dilated vessel-like metastatic glands in a background of marrow fibrosis *(A)*. Cytokeratin *(B)* and mucin *(C)* stains highlight the metastatic glandular structures.

Figure 2–17. Metastatic adenocarcinoma stimulating marrow fibrosis *(A)*. A high-power view *(B)* demonstrates infiltrating tumor cells, some of which show vacuolated cytoplasm (signet-ring pattern). Low- *(C)* and high-power *(D)* views of a cytokeratin stain depict numerous positive cells.

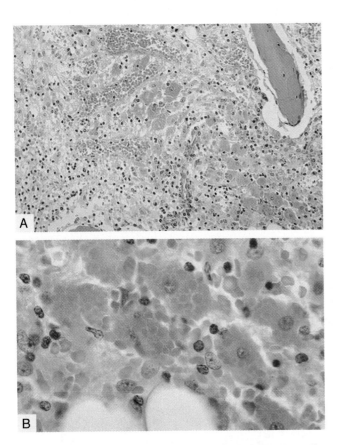

Figure 2–18. Bone marrow biopsy sections after chemotherapy and/or irradiation are markedly hypocellular and may demonstrate edema and increased number of histiocytes *(A)*. Some of the histiocytes may show evidence of hemophagocytosis *(B)*.

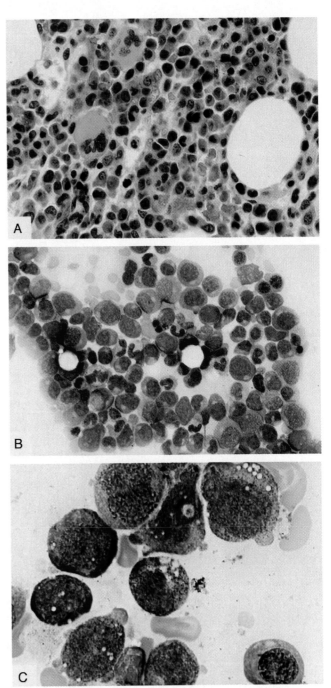

Figure 2–19. Bone marrow samples of granulocyte colony-stimulating factor (G-CSF)-treated patients may show increased cellularity *(A)*, myeloid left shift, and dysplastic changes *(B* and *C)*. The morphologic features may mimic myelodysplastic syndrome or even acute myelogenous leukemia. These changes will disappear shortly after withdrawal of the G-CSF therapy.

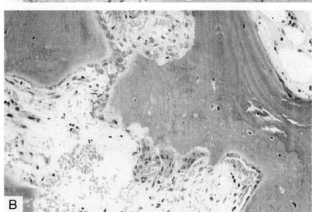

Figure 2–20. Bone marrow biopsies obtained from previous biopsy sites may show evidence of tissue repair, such as fibrosis and new bone formation. *A*, Osteoid deposits are surrounded by osteoblasts in a fibrotic bone marrow. *B*, Numerous osteoblasts and scattered osteoclasts are around the bone trabeculae.

ABNORMAL BONE MARROW AND BLOOD CYTOLOGY

Abnormal Erythroid Morphology

Abnormal morphology in erythroid precursors includes megaloblastic and dysplastic changes, cytoplasmic vacuolization, and the presence of ringed sideroblasts. Megaloblastic changes are frequent features of vitamin B12 and folate deficiencies, myelodysplastic syndromes (MDS), AZT therapy and chemotherapy (Figure 2–21). Dysplastic changes, such as nuclear/cytoplasmic maturation asynchrony, abnormal nuclear morphology, nuclear fragmentation, nuclear chromatin bridges, and multinucleation are observed in MDS, congenital dyserythropoietic anemia, megaloblastic anemia, erythroleukemia, and following chemotherapy.

A wide spectrum of red blood cell (RBC) abnormal morphology is observed in anemias and parasitic infections, which are best detected by blood smear examination. Examples are *anisocytosis* (variation in size), *poikilocytosis* (variation in shape), *microcytes, ovalocytes, stomatocytes, spherocytes, target cells, teardrops, frag-mented RBCs* (schistocytes), and cytoplasmic inclusions such as *Howell-Jolly bodies, Cabot's ring, basophilic stippling, Heinz bodies, Pappenheimer granules* (iron particles in RBCs), and *malaria* parasites (Figure 2–22).

Abnormal Leukocyte Morphology

Nuclear hypo- or hypersegmentation and abnormal cytoplasmic granulation are frequent morphologic abnormalities in the granulocytic series most commonly seen in MDS, myelogenous leukemias, G-CSF therapy, and chemotherapy. Hypersegmented neutrophils are also observed in megaloblastic anemia (see Figure 2–21).

Abnormal cytoplasmic inclusions include *Döhle inclusion bodies* (in infections, drug toxicity, burns), *Alder-Reilly anomaly* (in mucopolysaccharidosis), inclusions in *Chédiak-Higashi* syndrome, and *Auer rods* (in acute myelogenous leukemias) (Figure 2–23).

Foamy histiocytes are cells with lipid-containing vacuoles (Niemann-Pick disease, hypercholesterolemia, Wolman's disease, Tangier disease) (Figure 2–24). *Sea-blue histiocytes* show cytoplasmic ceroid-containing structures that stain sea-blue to blue-green with Wright's stain.

These cells are seen in a variety of hematologic disorders, such as MDS, chronic myeloproliferative disorders, hyperlipidemia, and hemolytic anemias (see Figure 2–24).

Prominent *hemophagocytosis* has been observed in association with viral and bacterial infections, hematologic malignancies, anticonvulsant drugs, and familial erythrophagocytic lymphohistiocytosis (see Figure 2–24).

In chronic and acute lymphoid leukemias and malignant lymphomas, the neoplastic cells often display abnormal morphology (Figure 2–25). Depending on the type of malignancy, the neoplastic cells may appear large or small with scant or abundant cytoplasm, regular or irregular nuclear border, fine or coarse nuclear chromatin, and presence or absence of prominent nucleoli. Reactive lymphocytes, frequently observed in viral infections, are large, pleomorphic cells with abundant cytoplasm and round or irregular nuclei. In multiple myeloma, bone marrow plasma cells are significantly increased in number and often show abnormal morphologic features (Figure 2–26). In plasma cell leukemia, plasma cells (≥20%) are found in the blood smears.

Abnormal Megakaryocytes and Platelets

Micromegakaryocytes are frequent findings in MDS and chronic myelogenous leukemia (CML). They appear as small mononuclear or binuclear megakaryocytes with variable amounts of hypogranular cytoplasm (Figure 2–27). Some micromegakaryocytes may show nuclear lobulation with two, three, or more lobules. Giant and multinuleated forms and megakaryocytic aggregates are

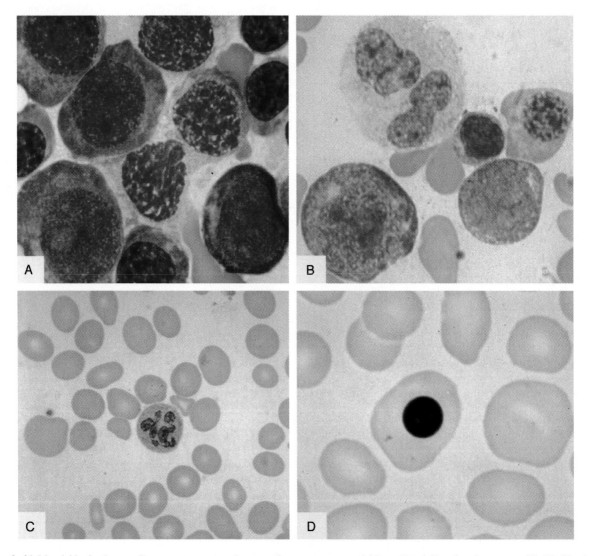

Figure 2–21 Megaloblastic changes. Bone marrow smears demonstrating numerous megaloblasts (*A* and *B*) and a giant neutrophil *(B)*. Blood smears showing macro-ovalocytes (*C* and *D*), a hypersegmented neutrophil *(C)*, and a late-stage nucleated red blood cell (rubricyte) with abundant hemoglobinized cytoplasm *(D)*. (From Naeim F: Pathology of Bone Marrow, 2nd ed. Baltimore, Williams & Wilkins, 1998, with permission.)

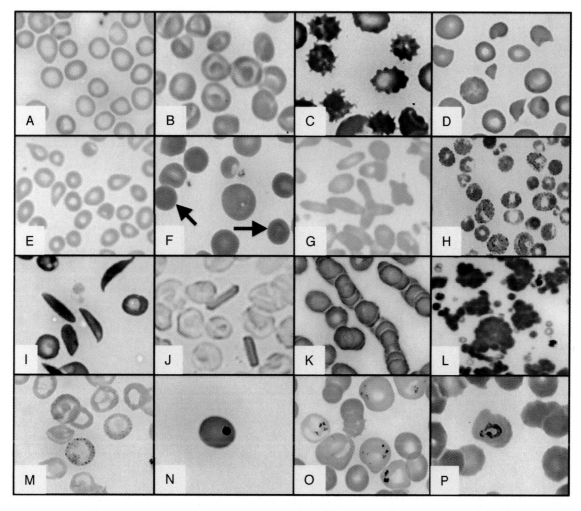

Figure 2–22. Abnormal red blood cell (RBC) morphology. Hypochromic erythrocytes *(A)* are seen in iron deficiency anemia and thalassemia. Target cells *(B)* are present in thalassemia, hemoglobinopathies, and liver disease. Echinocytes *(C)* are associated with uremia and pyruvate kinase deficiency. Schistocytes *(D)* are observed in microangiopathic hemolytic anemia. Teardrop forms *(E)* are frequently associated with myelofibrosis. Spherocytes *(F, arrows)* are present in hereditary spherocytosis and autoimmune hemolytic anemia. Elliptocytosis *(G)* is a hereditary disorder. Golf ball–like hemoglobin precipitates *(H)* are present in hemoglobin H disease. Sickle cells *(I)* and hemoglobin C crystals *(J)* are seen in sickle cell anemia and hemoglobin C disorder. RBC rouleaux formation *(K)* is associated with hypergammaglobunlinemia and hyperfibrinogenemia. RBC agglutination *(L)* is seen in cold hemagglutinin disease. Basophilic stippling *(M)* is a hallmark for lead poisoning. Howell-Jolly body *(N)* is present in megaloblastic anemia, in hemolytic anemia, and post-splenectomy. Pappenheimer granules (iron particles detected with Wright's stain) *(O)* are demonstrated in refractory anemia and thalassemia. Malaria parasites appear as RBC inclusions in ring *(P)* or other forms.

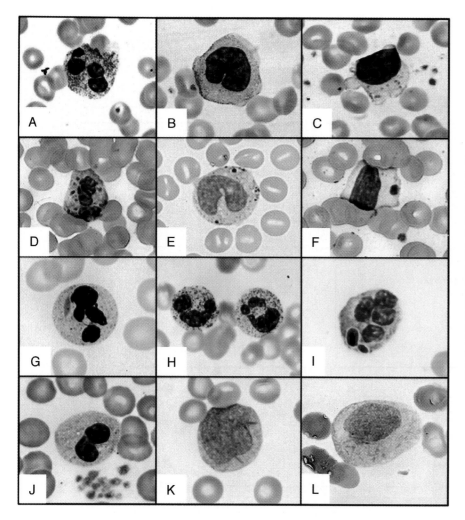

Figure 2–23. Abnormal leukocyte morphology. Alder-Reilly anomaly appears as numerous azurophilic cytoplasmic granules in neutrophils *(A)*, monocytes *(B)*, and lymphocytes *(C)* of patients with mucopolysaccharidosis. Cytoplasmic inclusions in Chédiak-Higashi syndrome are larger and fewer and are present in neutrophils *(D)*, monocytes *(E)*, and lymphocytes *(F)*. Döhle inclusion bodies *(G)* and toxic granulation *(H)* are found in neutrophils in conditions such as infections, drug toxicity, and burns. The presence of fungus *(I)* in the circulating neutrophils is a rare event. Hyposegmented neutrophils *(J)* are seen in Pelger-Huët anomaly as well as in myeloproliferative disorders and myelodysplastic syndromes. Auer rods *(K* and *L)* are noted in cells of acute myelogenous leukemia.

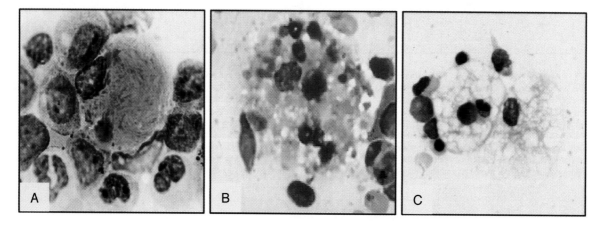

Figure 2–24. Sea-blue histiocytes *(A)* are frequently seen in myeloproliferative disorders and disorders that are associated with rapid or massive destruction of bone marrow cells. Increased numbers of macrophages with iron particles and/or phagocytic debris *(B)* are seen in iron overload and hemophagocytic syndromes. Foamy histiocytes *(C)* are present in a variety of storage disease/histiocytic disorders, such as Niemann-Pick disease, hypercholesterolemia, Wolman's disease, and Langerhans cell histiocytosis.

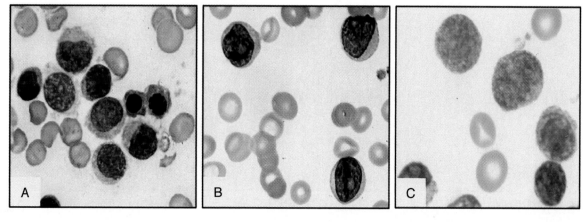

Figure 2–25. Examples of abnormal lymphocyte morphology. *A,* Bone marrow smear demonstrating large lymphoid cells with variable amounts of cytoplasm and cytoplasmic projections representing hairy cell leukemia. *B,* Blood smear depicting prolymphocytes with variable amounts of cytoplasm, coarse chromatin and prominent nucleolus in a patient with prolymphocytic leukemia. *C,* Blood smear depicting lymphoid cells with convoluted nuclei (Sézary cells) in a patient with cutaneous T-cell lymphoma.

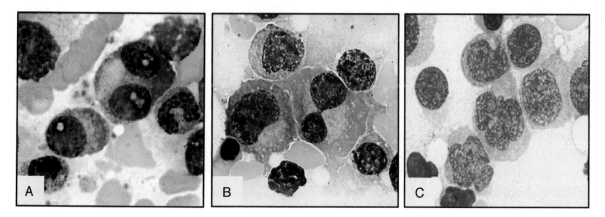

Figure 2–26. Atypical plasma cells in bone marrow smears of patients with plasma cell dyscrasia (*A, B* and *C*).

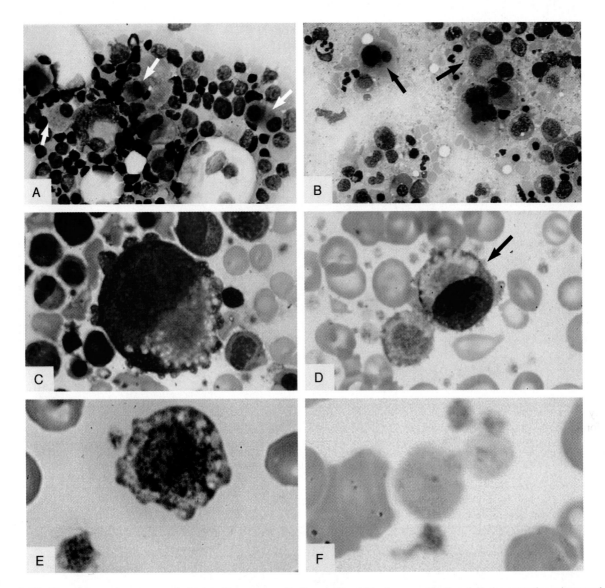

Figure 2–27. Abnormal megakaryocytes and platelets. Bone marrow (*A, B,* and *C*) and blood smears (*D, E,* and *F*) demonstrating micromegakaryocytes (*A, B,* and *D, arrows*), a dysplastic megakaryocyte with vacuolated cytoplasm *(C)*, giant platelets with abundant granules (*D* and *E*), and a giant platelet lacking granules *(F)*.

reported in chronic myeloproliferative disorders, MDS, and acute myeloid leukemias.

Giant platelets are seen in Bernard-Soulier syndrome, myeloproliferative disorders, and acute megakaryoblastic leukemia (AML-M7) (see Figure 2–27). Hypogranular platelets are seen in gray platelet syndrome (alpha granule deficiency), in acute megakaryoblastic leukemia, and sometimes in patients with hypersplenism (see Figure 2–27).

Selected References

Browne PM, Sharma OP, Salkin D: Bone marrow sarcoidosis. JAMA 240:2654, 1978.

Eid A, Carion W, Nystrom JS: Differential diagnoses of bone marrow granuloma. West J Med 164:510, 1996.

Howard MR, Kesteven PJL: Sea blue histiocytosis: A common abnormality of the bone marrow in myelodysplastic syndromes. J Clin Pathol 46:1030, 1993.

Kyle RA, Gertz MA, Greipp PR, et al: Long-term survival (10 years or more) in 30 patients with primary amyloidosis. Blood 93:1062, 1999.

Lee RE: Histiocytic diseases of bone marrow. Hematol Oncol Clin North Am 2:657, 1988.

Mais El D, Lim JY, Pollock WJ, et al: Bone marrow necrosis: An entity often overlooked. Ann Clin Lab Sci 18:109, 1988.

McCarthy DM: Fibrosis of the bone marrow: Content and causes. Br J Haematol 59:1, 1985.

Naeim F: Pathology of Bone Marrow, 2nd ed. Baltimore, Williams & Wilkins 1998, p 82.

Pantel K, Cote RJ, Fodstad O: Detection and clinical importance of micrometastatic disease. J Natl Cancer Inst 91:1113, 1999.

Seaman JP, Kjeldsberg CT, Linker A: Gelatinous transformation of the bone marrow. Hum Pathol 9:685, 1978.

Wickramasinghe SN: Blood and Bone Marrow, 3rd ed. London, Churchill Livingstone, 1986.

Wittels B: Bone marrow biopsy changes following chemotherapy for acute leukemia. Am J Surg Pathol 4:135, 1980.

CHAPTER 3

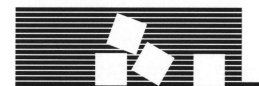

Myelodysplastic Syndromes

Myelodysplastic syndromes (MDS) or refractory anemias (RA) are clonal stem cell defects characterized by ineffective hematopoiesis and cytopenia. The defective stem cells may eventually undergo additional chromosomal abnormalities, resulting in transformation of MDS to acute leukemia.

MDS is either primary (etiology unknown) or therapy related (history of radiation or chemotherapy). The frequency of marrow fibrosis, chromosome abnormality, and transformation to acute leukemia is higher in the therapy-related MDS (T-MDS) than in the primary MDS.

Myelodysplastic changes, similar to MDS, have been observed in a variety of conditions, such as endocrinopathies, autoimmune disorders, human immunodeficiency virus (HIV) infection, and following granulocyte colony-stimulating factor (G-CSF) therapy. The dysplastic changes in these conditions, unlike MDS, are not clonal, and therefore, are not associated with cytogenetic abnormalities.

Bone marrow and blood examination of MDS patients usually reveals a variety of abnormal morphology and dysplastic changes, including:

Topographical rearrangements, such as peritrabecular localization of erythroid cells and megakaryocytes, and localization of immature myeloid aggregates away from bone trabeculae (abnormal localization of immature precursors [ALIP]) (Figures 3–1 and 3–2).

Focal or diffuse bone marrow fibrosis, and the presence of edema and inflammatory cells.

Abnormal erythroid morphology, such as megaloblastic changes, macrocytosis, anisopoikilocytosis, basophilic stippling, and the presence of ringed sideroblasts (Figure 3–3).

Dysgranulocytopoiesis, such as abnormal cell size, cytoplasmic hypo- or hypergranulation, and nuclear hypo- or hypersegmentation (Figures 3–4 and 3–5).

Megakaryocytic dysplasia and abnormal platelets, such as the presence of micromegakaryocytes and giant platelets (Figure 3–6).

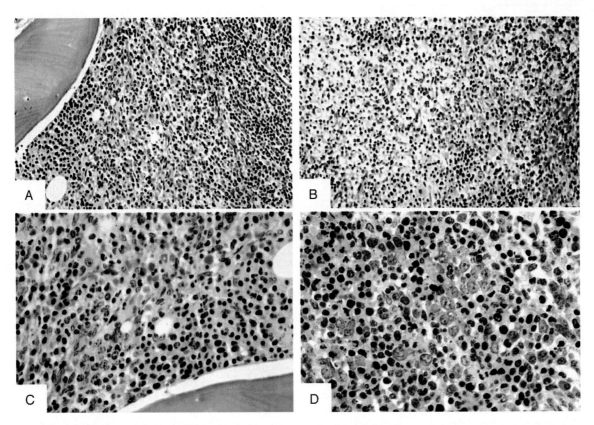

Figure 3–1. Bone marrow biopsy sections from a patient with myelodysplastic syndrome demonstrating hypercellularity with the presence of lymphoid aggregate (*A*), areas of edema (*B*), peritrabecular localization of the erythroid precursors (*C*), and the presence of small clusters of immature cells (*D*).

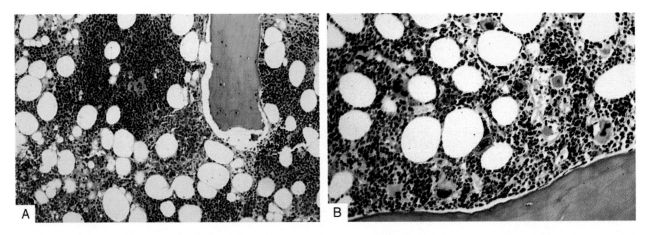

Figure 3–2. Bone marrow biopsy sections from a patient with therapy-related myelodysplastic syndrome demonstrating marked erythroid preponderance *(A)* with localization of the erythroid precursors and megakaryocytes close to the bone trabeculae *(B)*.

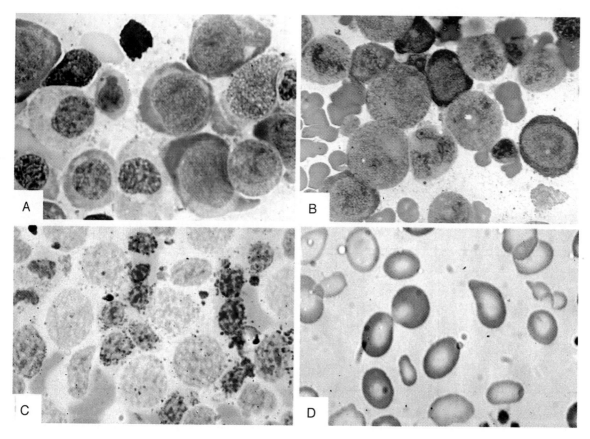

Figure 3–3. Abnormal erythropoiesis. Bone marrow smears showing megaloblastic changes (*A* and *B*) and the presence of numerous ringed sideroblasts by the Prussian blue stain (*C*). Blood smear demonstrating aniso-poikilocytosis with macro-ovalocytes and schistocytes (*D*).

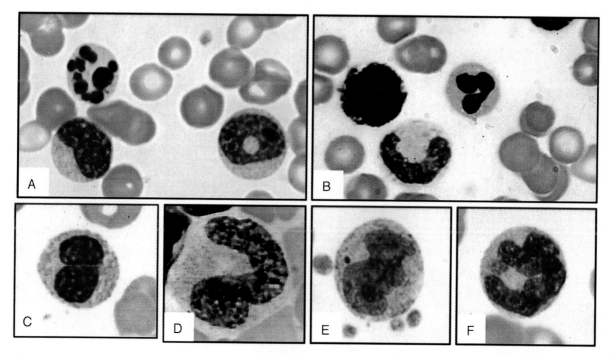

Figure 3–4. Abnormal granulocytopoiesis. A variety of abnormal myeloid cells have been observed in patients with myelodysplastic syndrome, such as hypersegmentation (*A* and *F*), hypogranulation (*B*), hyposegmentation (*C*), giant forms (*D* and *E*), and cells with ring-formed (doughnut-like) nucleus (*A*).

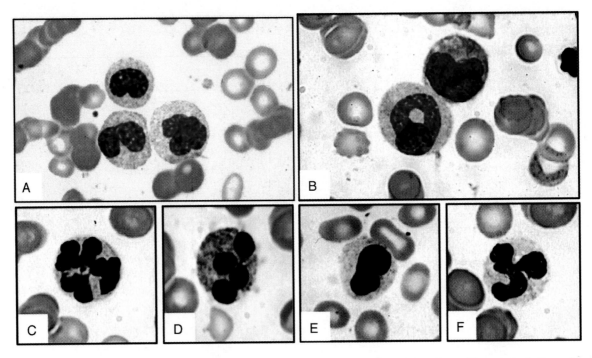

Figure 3–5. Abnormal granulocytopoiesis. A variety of abnormal myeloid cells have been observed in patients with myelodysplastic syndrome, such as hyposegmentation or hypersegmentation of the granulocytes (*A* and *C*), ringed-form nuclei (*B*), hypogranulation (*B*, *E*, and *F*), and hypergranulation (*D*).

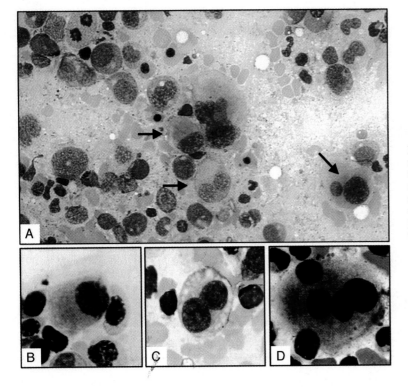

Figure 3–6. Abnormal megakaryocytes. The most prominent dysplastic change in the megakaryocytic lineage is the presence of micromegakaryocytes (*A*, *arrows; B* and *C*). Micromegakaryocytes appear as small mononuclear and binuclear megakaryocytes, or as megakaryocytes with a bilobed nucleus. Larger megakaryocytes may also display abnormal morphology, such as the presence of several separated nuclei (*D*).

CLASSIFICATION

The original classification of MDS, proposed by the French-American-British (FAB) Cooperative Group, included five major categories: refractory anemia, refractory anemia with ringed sideroblasts, refractory anemia with excess blasts, chronic myelomonocytic leukemia, and refractory anemia with excess blasts in transformation. Later, a few more entities, such as chronic myelomonocytc leukemia in transformation, were added to the list. A new classification has been recently proposed by the World Health Organization (WHO). This classification includes two major categories: (1) MDS, featuring dysplasia and cytopenia; and (2) syndromes that display features of both MDS and myeloproliferative disorders, such as the combination of dysplasia and cytosis. These two major categories are listed in Table 3–1 and are briefly discussed below.

Refractory Anemia

RA is a dyserythropoietic process which leads to reticulocytopenia and anemia. Bone marrow is normo- or hypercellular with erythroid hyperplasia and often increased iron stores (Figure 3–7). Ringed sideroblasts are absent or rare (<15% of nucleated red cells). Erythrocytes may show anisopoikilocytosis and/or macrocytosis. Granulocytic and megakaryocytic dysplasia is insignificant and there is no evidence of increased myeloblasts. Occasionally, instead of anemia, granulocytopenia or thrombocytopenia is present. In such cases, bone marrow often shows dysplastic changes in the precursor cells that are associated with cytopenia.

Refractory Anemia With Ringed Sideroblasts

The characteristics of refractory anemia with ringed sideroblasts (RARS) are similar to that of RA except that greater than 15% of the bone marrow nucleated red cells are ringed sideroblasts (Figure 3–8). RA and RARS have a longer median survival and lower incidence of progression to acute leukemia than the other types of MDS.

Refractory Cytopenia With Multilineage Dysplasia

This condition is associated with the presence of dysplastic changes in two or more hematopoietic lineages (Figures 3–9 and 3–10). Myeloblasts are less than 5% of the bone marrow cells.

Refractory Anemia With Excess Blasts

Refractory anemia with excess blasts (RAEB) is associated with cytopenia affecting two or more of the hematopoietic lines. Bone marrow is usually hyper- or normocellular, but rarely hypocellular, with dysplastic changes, myeloid left shift, and increased myeloblasts (Figures 3–11 and 3–12). Myeloblasts range from over 5% to less than 20% in the bone marrow and less than 5% in the peripheral blood. Auer rods are not seen. Ringed sideroblasts may be present but are usually less than 15% of the nucleated red cells.

Refractory Anemia With Excess Blasts in Transformation

Morphologic features of refractory anemia with excess blasts in transformation (RAEB-T) are similar to those of RAEB except for higher percent of blast cells in bone marrow and/or peripheral blood (Figure 3–13). Blasts are between 20% and 30% of the nucleated cells in the bone marrow and greater than 5% of the leukocytes in the peripheral blood. Auer rods may be present. RAEB-T, a subtype in FAB classification, has been eliminated from the WHO classification because of its similarity in prognosis with AML. According to the WHO guidelines, the required number of blasts for the diagnosis of AML is ≥20% (see Chapter 5).

Chronic Myelomonocytic Leukemia

Chronic myelomonocytic leukemia (CMML) manifests morphologic features shared in both MDS and myeloproliferative disorders. Bone marrow is usually hypercellular and demonstrates myeloid left shift with increased immature myelomonocytic cells (Figures 3–14 to 3–16). The total percentage of blasts ranges from more than 5% to less than 20%. Blood shows absolute monocytosis of greater than 1,000/μL with less than 5% blasts (see Figure 3–14). Identification of the monocytic precursors in the marrow may require cytochemical stains (nonspecific esterase, lysozyme) and/or immunophenotypic studies (CD14, CD64, CD68) (see Figures 3–14 and 3–15).

Chronic Myelomonocytic Leukemia in Transformation

Chronic myelomonocytic leukemia in transformation (CMML-T) is similar to that of CMML except for a higher percent of myeloblasts and monocytic precursors (monoblasts and promonocytes) in bone marrow and/or peripheral blood. The blasts/promonocytes are between 20% and 29% of the bone marrow cells and greater than 5% of the leukocytes in the peripheral blood. This entity, similar to RAEB-T, is not included in the WHO classification, and is considered as a variant of AML (see Chapter 5).

Juvenile Myelomonocytic Leukemia

Juvenile myelomonocytic leukemia (JMML) (formerly referred to as juvenile chronic myeloid leukemia) is a rare myelodysplastic/myeloproliferative disorder of infancy and childhood with morphologic features similar to CMML (see Figure 3–14). However, affected patients frequently demonstrate cutaneous manifestations (such as eczema and xanthoma), elevated levels of fetal hemoglobin, and low expression of the red blood cell I antigen. This disorder shares many features with infantile monosomy 7 syndrome.

Atypical Chronic Myelogenous Leukemia

Atypical chronic myelogenous leukemia (aCML) is very similar to CML except for the lack of Ph[1] [t(9;22), bcr-abl rearrangement]. This disorder is usually associated with marked myeloid dysplasia and the presence of immature myeloid cells in peripheral blood. Unlike in CML, basophilia is often not present in aCML.

Other Related Disorders

Hypocellular MDS

Approximately 10% to 15% of the MDS patients demonstrate a hypocellular bone marrow ($<20-25\%$ cellularity). The majority of these cases fall into the category of T-MDS (Figure 3–17).

MDS With Fibrosis

Mild to moderate focal marrow fibrosis is a frequent finding in MDS, particularly in T-MDS. Marked marrow fibrosis has been reported in over 50% of the T-MDS and 10% to 15% of the primary MDS cases.

Nonclonal MDS

Several conditions, such as autoimmune disorders, HIV infection, nonhematologic malignancies, heavy metal toxicity, chemotherapy, and irradiation, are sometimes associated with nonclonal (normal karyotype) myelodysplastic changes. These changes are usually reversible upon elimination of the primary cause.

Text continued on page 42

Table 3–1

PROPOSED WHO CLASSIFICATION OF MYELODYSPLASTIC SYNDROMES AND RELATED DISORDERS*

I. Myelodysplastic Syndromes
Refractory anemia (RA)
Refractory anemia with ringed sideroblasts (RARS)
Refractory cytopenia with multilineage dysplasia (RCMD)
Refractory anemia with excess blasts (RAEB)
5q-syndrome
Myelodysplastic syndrome, unclassified

II. Myelodysplastic/Myeloproliferative Disorders
Chronic myelomonocytic leukemia (CMML)
Juvenile myelomonocytic leukemia (JMML)
Atypical chronic myelogenous leukemia (aCML)

*Myelodysplastic syndromes are either primary *(de novo)* or therapy related.
Note: Entities such as RAEB-T and CMML-T are eliminated from this classification and are considered variants of AML. According to the WHO guidelines, the minimum required number of blasts for the diagnosis of AML is 20%.

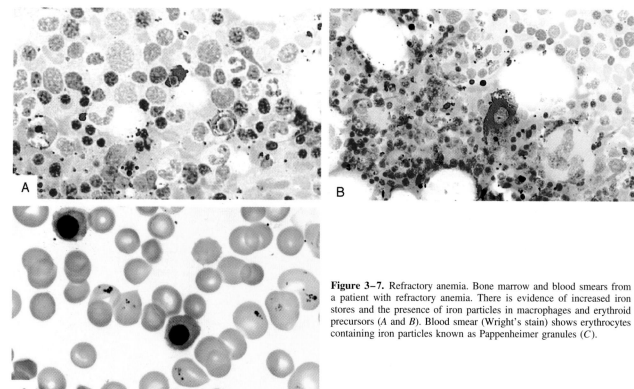

Figure 3-7. Refractory anemia. Bone marrow and blood smears from a patient with refractory anemia. There is evidence of increased iron stores and the presence of iron particles in macrophages and erythroid precursors (*A* and *B*). Blood smear (Wright's stain) shows erythrocytes containing iron particles known as Pappenheimer granules (*C*).

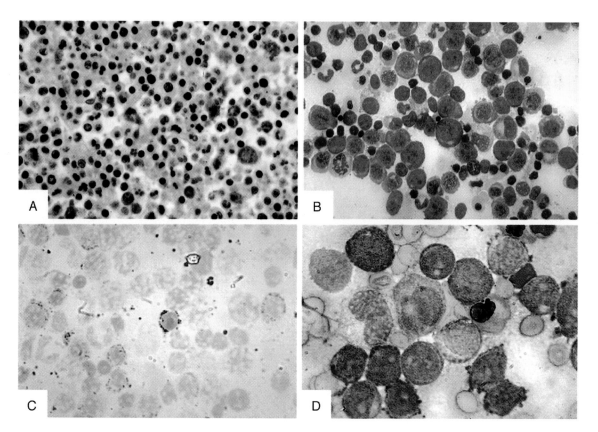

Figure 3-8. Refractory anemia with ringed sideroblasts. Bone marrow biopsy section (*A*) and marrow smear (*B*) show marked erythroid preponderance with megaloblastic features, and the iron stain demonstrates numerous ringed sideroblasts (*C*). Dysplastic erythroid cells may show coarse, periodic acid-Schiff (PAS)-positive cytoplasmic granules (*D*).

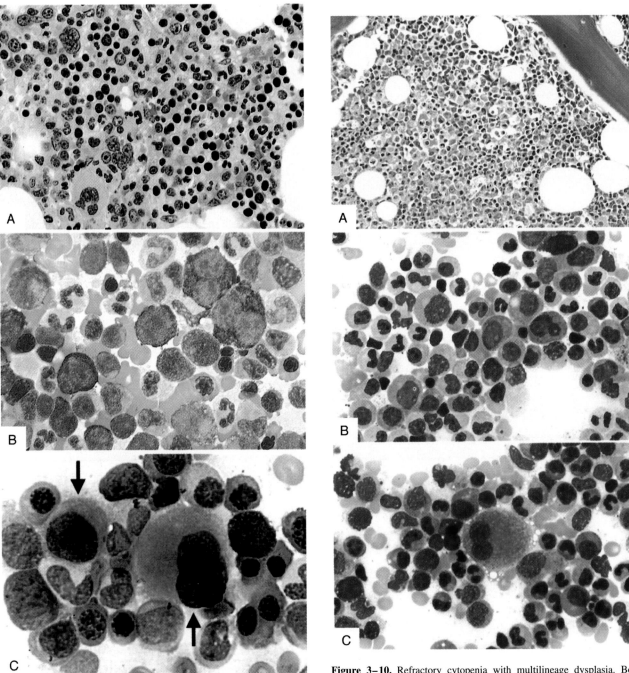

Figure 3–9. Refractory cytopenia with multilineage dysplasia. Bone marrow biopsy section (A) is hypercellular and shows erythroid preponderance. Bone marrow smears demonstrate dysplastic erythropoiesis (B) and micromegakaryocytes (C, arrows).

Figure 3–10. Refractory cytopenia with multilineage dysplasia. Bone marrow biopsy section (A) is hypercellular and shows myeloid preponderance. Bone marrow smears demonstrate dysplastic myelopoiesis with hyposegmented neutrophils and hypogranular myeloid cells (B and C). A micromegakaryocyte is demonstrated (C).

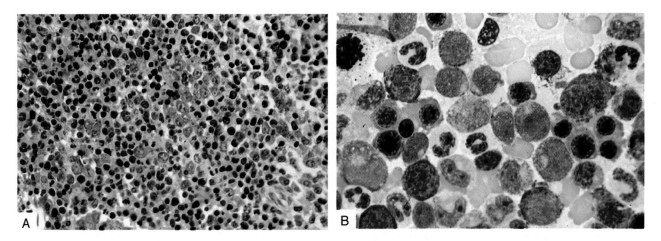

Figure 3–11. Refractory anemia with excess blasts (RAEB). Bone marrow biopsy section (*A*) is hypercellular and shows erythroid preponderance and clusters of immature myeloid cells (atypical localization of immature precursors [ALIP]). Bone marrow smear (*B*) demonstrates increased immature myeloid cells and myeloblasts.

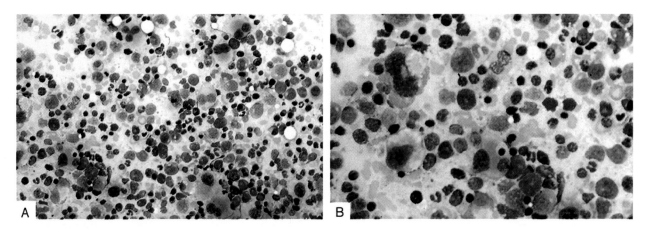

Figure 3–12. Refractory anemia with excess blasts (RAEB). Low- (*A*) and high-power (*B*) views of a bone marrow smear demonstrate numerous micromegakaryocytes and increased myeloblasts.

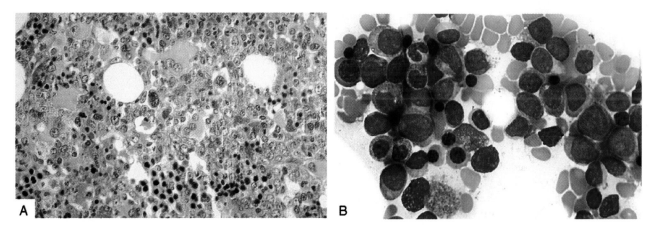

Figure 3–13. Bone marrow biopsy section (*A*) demonstrates clusters of blast cells, and bone marrow smear (*B*) displays increased numbers of myeloblasts (the differential count showed 24% blasts). These features are consistent with RAEB-T based on the FAB classification, and AML according to the WHO guidelines.

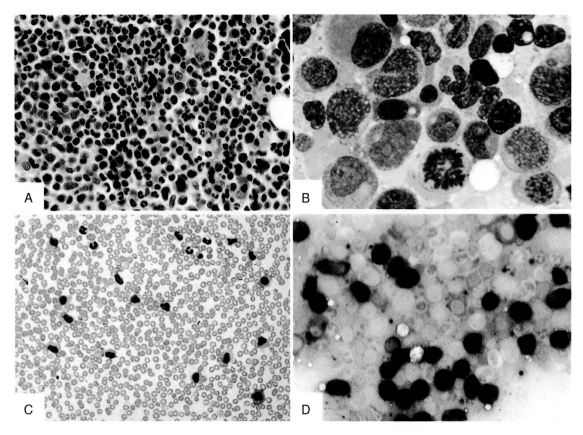

Figure 3–14. Chronic myelomonocytic leukemia (CMML). Bone marrow biopsy section (*A*) is hypercellular with increased number of immature cells. Bone marrow smear (*B*) demonstrates myeloid left shift with myeloblasts and immature monocytes (monoblasts, promonocytes). There is evidence of peripheral blood monocytosis (*C*), and numerous cells in the bone marrow smear show positive reaction with nonspecific esterase stain (*D*).

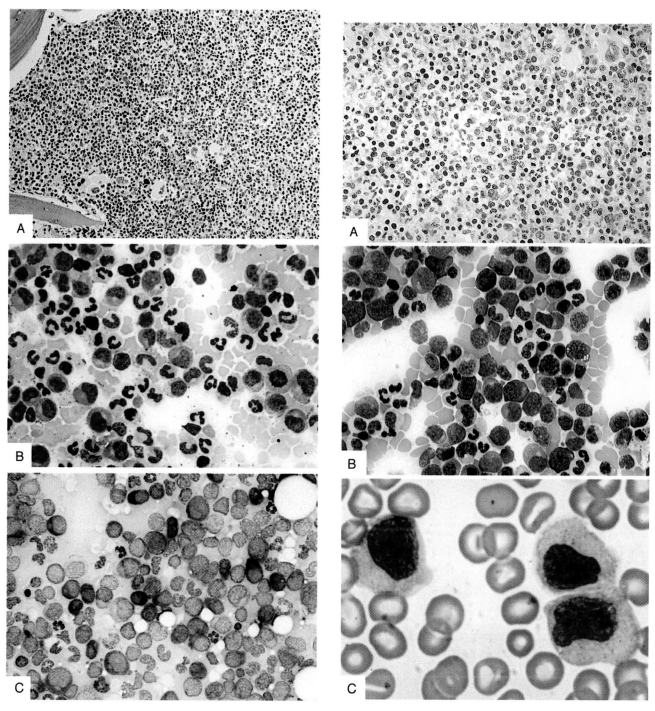

Figure 3–15. Chronic myelomonocytic leukemia (CMML). Bone marrow biopsy section (*A*) is hypercellular with increased number of immature cells. Bone marrow smear (*B*) demonstrates myeloid left shift (myeloblasts, monoblasts, and promonocytes). Numerous immature cells in the bone marrow smear show positive reaction with the nonspecific esterase stain (*C*).

Figure 3–16. Chronic myelomonocytic leukemia (CMML). Bone marrow biopsy section (*A*) is hypercellular with increased number of immature cells. Bone marrow smear (*B*) demonstrates myeloid left shift with increased myeloblasts, monoblasts, and promonocytes. There is evidence of peripheral blood monocytosis (*C*).

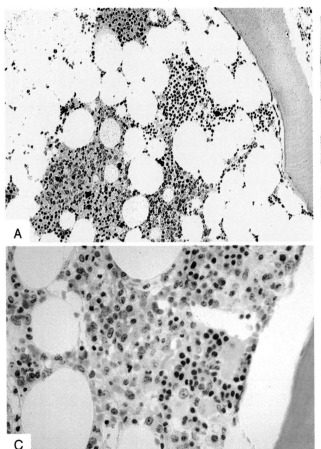

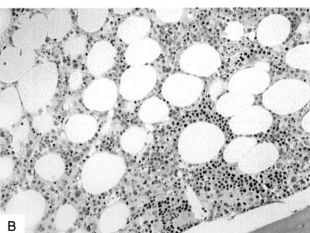

Figure 3–17. Hypocellular myelodysplastic syndrome (MDS): Low-, intermediate-, and high-power views (*A*, *B*, and *C*, respectively) of a bone marrow biopsy section from a patient with therapy-related myelodysplastic syndrome demonstrating a hypocellular marrow with peritrabecular localization of the erythroid cells and myeloid left shift.

CYTOGENETIC ABNORMALITIES

The incidence of cytogenetic abnormalities in MDS ranges from 40% to 98%. The higher figures belong to the T-MDS. The most common chromosomal aberrations in primary MDS are 5q- (Figure 3–18), trisomy 8 (Figure 3–19), and monosomy 7. The most frequent cytogenetic abnormalities in T-MDS are monosomy 7, 5q-, and monosomy 5 (Table 3–2).

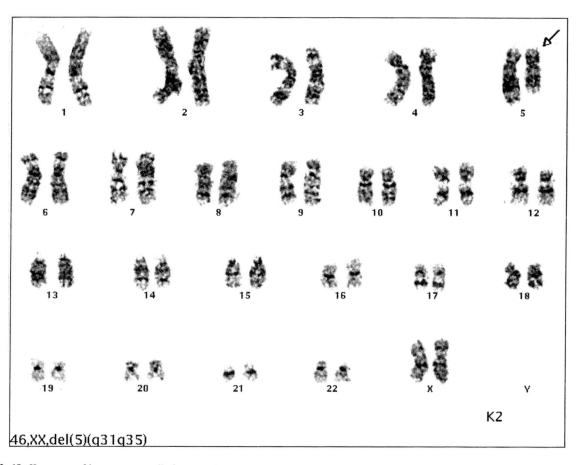

46,XX,del(5)(q31q35)

Figure 3–18. Karyotype of bone marrow cells from a patient with MDS demonstrating deletion of the long arm of chromosome 5 (5q-). (Courtesy of Nagesh Rao, Ph.D., Department of Pathology and Laboratory Medicine, UCLA School of Medicine.)

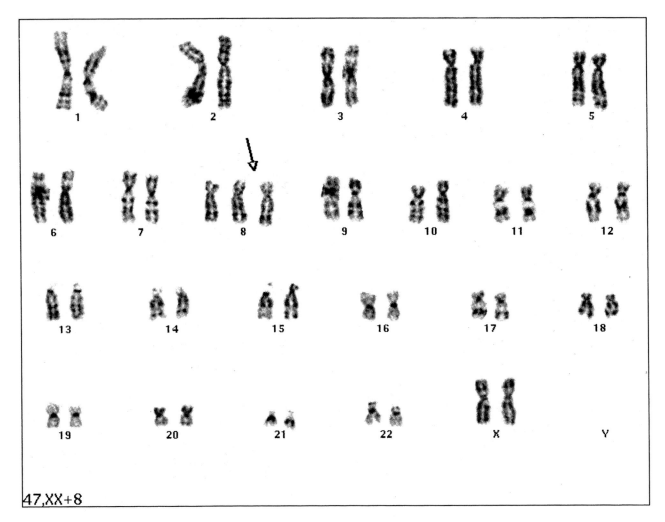

47,XX+8

Figure 3–19. Karyotype of bone marrow cells from a patient with MDS demonstrating an extra chromosome 8 (trisomy 8). (Courtesy of Nagesh Rao, Ph.D., Department of Pathology and Laboratory Medicine, UCLA School of Medicine.)

Table 3–2
MOST FREQUENT CYTOGENETIC ABNORMALITIES IN
PATIENTS WITH MYELODYSPLASTIC SYNDROMES

Primary		Therapy-Related	
Aberrations	*Incidence (%)*	*Aberrations*	*Incidence (%)*
5q-	27	−7	41
+8	19	5q-	28
−7	15	−5	11
der(11q)	7	der(21q)	9
−5	5	7q-	8
der(12p)	5	+8	8
-Y	5	der(12p)	8
20q-	2	t(1;7)	7

Adapted from Heim S: Cytogenetic findings in primary and secondary MDS. Leuk Res 16:43, 1992.

CLINICAL ASPECTS

Primary MDS are uncommon under the age of 50 years, whereas T-MDS may affect patients at any age. T-MDS usually appear 4 to 5 years following chemotherapy and/or irradiation. Patients may be asymptomatic or may demonstrate mild to severe symptoms related to one or several cytopenias. A number of conditions are reported in association with poor prognosis, such as multilineage dysplasia, increased blasts, chromosome 7 aberrations, or presence of two or more cytogenetic abnormalities. Normal cytogenetic results, 5q- alone, 20q- alone, and -Y alone have been associated with favorable prognosis.

DIFFERENTIAL DIAGNOSIS

A broad spectrum of hematologic disorders may demonstrate dysplastic changes in the bone marrow and, therefore, should be considered in the differential diagnosis of MDS.

Megaloblastic anemia may mimic RA and RARS. However, in megaloblastic anemia, folate or vitamin B12 levels are low and there is a normal karyotype.

Congenital dyserythropoietic anemias are inherited disorders with marked dyserythropoiesis (see Chapter 14). Erythrocytes may demonstrate a positive reaction in the serum acid test. Ringed sideroblasts are usually absent. Myeloid series and megakaryocytes are unremarkable, and cytogenetic studies are normal.

MDS with fibrosis should be distinguished from primary myelofibrosis and acute leukemias that are associated with bone marrow fibrosis. The distinction is sometimes difficult due to the frequent failure of bone marrow aspiration (dry tap) because of the marrow fibrosis. Marked splenomegaly and the presence of leukoerythroblastic pattern in blood smear (presence of immature myeloid cells and nucleated red blood cells) are in favor of a primary myelofibrosis. The presence of increased blasts in bone marrow sections or blood smears is in favor of acute leukemia.

Differential diagnosis of RAEB from acute myelogenous leukemia is sometimes problematic, particularly when the decision is based on the number of type II and III myeloblasts. Multilineage dysplasia is the characteristic feature of RAEB, whereas it is less frequent in acute leukemias. In erythroleukemia the myeloid:erythroid (M:E) ratio is less than 1, and the percent blast cells in the nonerythroid bone marrow cells is 30 or above.

Conditions under the category of myelodysplastic/myeloproliferative disorders (see Table 3–1), such as CMML and JMML may show significant overlapping features with chronic myelogenous leukemia in chronic or accelerated phase. However, CMML and JMML are negative for Ph¹/abl-bcr, and show a normal or elevated leukocyte alkaline phosphatase (LAP) score.

Transient myeloproliferative disorder in Down syndrome observed in neonates may mimic RAEB or acute myelogenous leukemia (AML). This disorder usually disappears spontaneously within 4 to 6 weeks, but occasionally may progress to AML (see Chapter 12).

Selected References

Aricò M, Biondi A, Pui CH: Juvenile myelomonocytic leukemia. Blood 90:479, 1997.
Bartl R, Frisch B, Baumgar R: Morphologic classification of the myelodysplastic syndromes (MDS): Combined utilization of bone marrow aspirates and trephine biopsies. Leuk Res 16:15, 1992.
Bennett JM, Sandberg AA, Third MIC Cooperative Study Group (1987): Morphologic, immunologic, and cytogenetic (MIC) working classification of the primary myelodysplastic syndromes and therapy-related myelodysplasias and leukemias. Cancer Genet Cytogenet 32:1, 1988.
Goasguen JE, Bennett JM: Classification and morphologic features of the myelodysplastic syndromes. Semin Oncol 19:4, 1992.
Harris NL, Jaffe ES, Diebold J, et al: The World Health Organization classification of hematological malignancies. Report of the Clinical Advisory Committee Meeting. Airlie House, Virginia, November 1997. Mod Pathol 13:193, 2000.
Heaney ML, Golde DW: Myelodysplasia. N Engl J Med 340:1649, 1999.
Kouides PA, Bennett JM: Morphology and classification of myelodysplastic syndromes and their pathologic variants. Semin Hematol 33: 95, 1996.
Levine EG, Bloomfield CD: Leukemias and myelodysplastic syndromes secondary to drug, radiation, and environmental exposure. Semin Oncol 19:47, 1992.
Mangi MH, Mufti GJ: Primary myelodysplastic syndromes: Diagnostic and prognostic significance of immunohistochemical assessment of bone marrow biopsies. Blood 79:198, 1992.
Mangi MH, Salisbury JR, Mufti GJ, et al: Abnormal localization of immature precursors (ALIP) in the bone marrow of myelodysplastic syndromes; current state of knowledge and future directions. Leuk Res 15:627, 1991.
Martiat P, Michaux JL, Rodhain J, et al: Philadelphia-Negative (Ph−) chronic myeloid leukemia (CML): comparison with Ph+ CML and chronic myelomonocytic leukemia. Blood 78:205, 1991.
Michaux J-L, Martiat P: Chronic myelomonocytic leukemia (CMML)— A myelodysplastic or myeloproliferative syndrome? Leuk Lymph 9: 35, 1993.
Naeim F: Pathology of Bone Marrow. Baltimore, Williams & Wilkins 1997, p 140.
Niemeyer CM, Arico M, Basso G, et al: Chronic myelomonocytic leukemia in childhood: A retrospective analysis of 110 cases. European Working Group on Myelodysplastic Syndromes in Childhood (EWOG-MDS). Blood 89:3534, 1997.
Passmore SJ, Hann IM, Stiller CA, et al: Pediatric myelodysplasia; a study of 68 children and a new prognostic scoring system. Blood 85: 1742, 1995.
Rosenbloom B, Schreck R, Koefller HP: Therapy-related myelodysplastic syndromes. Hematol Oncol Clin North Am 6:707, 1992.
Vallespí T, Imbert M, Mecucci C, et al: Diagnosis, classification, and cytogenetics of myelodysplastic syndromes. Haematologica 83:258, 1998.
Vardiman JW, Head D: Society for Hematopathology: The myelodysplastic syndromes and related disorders. Mod Pathol 12:101, 1999.
Verhoef GEG, Pittaluga S, De Wolf-Peeters C: FAB classification of myelodysplastic syndromes: Merits and controversies. Ann Hematol 71:3, 1995.
Winfield DA, Polacarz SV: Bone marrow histology 3: Value of bone marrow core biopsy in acute leukemia, myelodysplastic syndromes, and chronic myelogenous leukemia. J Clin Pathol 45:855, 1992.

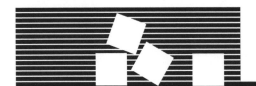

CHAPTER 4

Chronic Myeloproliferative Disorders

Chronic myeloproliferative disorders (CMPD) are the result of clonal proliferation of defective multipotent bone marrow stem cells. The stem cell defect in CMPD, unlike MDS, does not lead to cytopenia. Instead, CMPD are associated with hyperplasia of one or more hematopoietic lineages, bone marrow hypercellularity, and elevated counts of hematopoietic cells in the peripheral blood (cytosis). CMPD represent a preleukemic or chronic leukemic phase that may eventually evolve into an acute leukemia.

Traditionally, four major types of CMPD have been described: polycythemia vera, essential thrombocythemia, agnogenic myeloid metaplasia with myelofibrosis, and chronic myelogenous leukemia. These entities share many clinicopathologic features, such as splenomegaly and hepatomegaly, bone marrow hypercellularity, increased and/or dysplastic megakaryocytes, and bone marrow fibrosis. Teardrop-shaped erythrocytes, basophilia, and giant platelets are also frequently observed.

POLYCYTHEMIA VERA

Polycythemia vera *(polycythemia rubra vera)* (PV) is characterized by absolute erythrocytosis, and varying degrees of leukocytosis, thrombocytosis, and splenomegaly. The criteria proposed by the Polycythemia Vera Study Group consist of two major sets of laboratory findings: categories A and B (Table 4–1). The diagnosis of PV is made if all three laboratory findings of category A are present, or if parameters 1 and 2 from category A plus any two parameters from category B are present.

In the active erythropoietic phase of the disease, bone marrow is hypercellular and displays erythroid hyperplasia (Figure 4–1), often with increase in the granulocytic precursors and megakaryocytes (Figure 4–2). However, it should be emphasized that the bone marrow morphology is widely variable in PV and offers no pathognomonic diagnostic features (see Figure 4–2). Blood smears often show bluish polychromatophilic red blood cells (RBCs; see Figure 4–1), elevated leukocyte alkaline phosphatase (LAP), basophilia, and large platelets.

Approximately 15% of the PV patients develop a condition very similar to agnogenic myeloid metaplasia (see below). This condition, known *as postpolycythemic myeloid metaplasia* (PPMM) or *spent phase*, is characterized by normalization of the red cell mass, bone marrow fibrosis, leukoerythroblastic peripheral blood, and increased splenomegaly. The risk of acute leukemia is higher in those patients who develop PPMM or receive ^{32}P or alkylating agents.

Cytogenetic abnormalities are reported in about 15% to 30% of the patients with no history of chemotherapy, and over 50% of patients who have received chemotherapy. The most frequent chromosomal aberrations in PV are trisomy 8, trisomy 9, add(1q), 20q-, 5q-, 11q-, 13q-, 1p-, and loss of Y chromosome.

Clinical Aspects

The most common symptoms and signs are headache, weakness, pruritus, dizziness, hepatosplenomegaly, and engorged retinal veins. Most PV patients are over the age of 50 years.

Differential Diagnosis

Differential diagnosis includes relative polycythemia (decreased plasma volume), erythrocytosis secondary to hypoxemia, and elevated levels of tumor-induced erythropoietin (cerebellar hemangioma, renal cell carcinoma, hepatocellular carcinoma). Absolute erythrocytosis associated with increased release of erythropoietin is called *secondary* polycythemia. The PPMM phase of the disease should be distinguished from the cellular phase of myelofibrosis with extramedullary hematopoiesis.

Table 4–1
CRITERIA FOR THE DIAGNOSIS OF POLYCYTHEMIA VERA*

Category A

Increased erythrocyte volume of >36 μL/kg in males and >32 μL/kg in females
Arterial saturation of >92%
Splenomegaly

Category B

Platelet count > 400,000/μL
Leukocytosis with WBC > 12,000/μL (in the absence of fever or infection)
Elevated leukocyte alkaline phosphatase (LAP) score (in the absence of fever or infection)
Serum vitamin B_{12} level > 900 pg/μL or unbound vitamin B_{12}–binding capacity of >2200 pg/μL

*The diagnosis of polycythemia vera (PV) is made if all three laboratory findings of category A are present or if parameters 1 and 2 from category A with any two parameters of category B are demonstrated; proposed by the Polycythemia Vera Study Group.

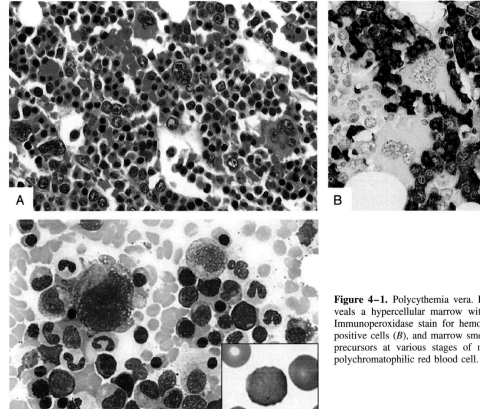

Figure 4–1. Polycythemia vera. Bone marrow biopsy section (*A*) reveals a hypercellular marrow with marked erythroid preponderance. Immunoperoxidase stain for hemoglobin A shows several clusters of positive cells (*B*), and marrow smear demonstrates numerous erythroid precursors at various stages of maturation (*C*). The inset shows a polychromatophilic red blood cell.

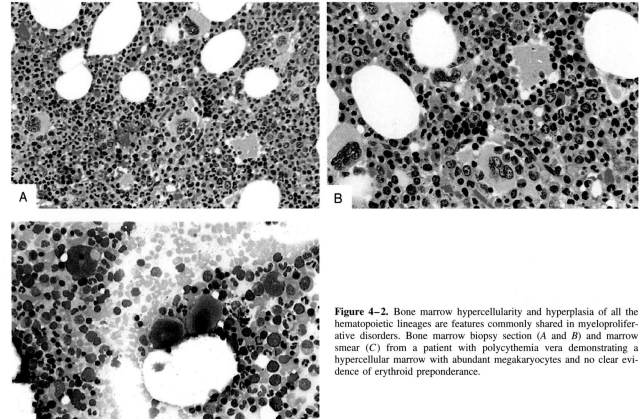

Figure 4–2. Bone marrow hypercellularity and hyperplasia of all the hematopoietic lineages are features commonly shared in myeloproliferative disorders. Bone marrow biopsy section (*A* and *B*) and marrow smear (*C*) from a patient with polycythemia vera demonstrating a hypercellular marrow with abundant megakaryocytes and no clear evidence of erythroid preponderance.

ESSENTIAL THROMBOCYTHEMIA

Essential thrombocythemia (ET) or *primary thrombocythemia* is characterized by persistent megakaryocytosis and thrombocytemia (>600,000/μL). For the establishment of the diagnosis of ET, other possible causes of thrombocythemia, such as other types of myeloproliferative disorders and iron deficiency anemia, should be ruled out. Bone marrow fibrosis, splenomegaly, and leukoerythroblastic reactions are absent or rare in ET (Table 4–2).

The bone marrow morphology is highly variable (Figures 4–3 to 4–6). In most instances, bone marrow is hypercellular and there is evidence of marked megakaryocytosis. Large megakaryocytes with hyperlobulated nuclei are present in clusters or are diffusely dispersed, and some are in close proximity of the bone trabeculae. Emperipolesis (internalization of hematopoietic cells) is often evident (see Figure 4–3).

Blood smears show marked increase in platelets with giant and/or atypical forms (see Figure 4–6). Platelet aggregates and megakaryocytic fragments may be present.

Aproximately 5% of ET patients may show abnormal chromosomes, such as del(13q) and del(21q).

Clinical Aspects

ET patients are usually over 50 years of age and often show abnormal platelet function leading to thrombotic or hemorrhagic complications. Splenomegaly may be present. Unexplained thrombocytosis without clinical symptoms is the only finding in a significant proportion of patients with ET.

Differential Diagnosis

Differential diagnosis includes other forms of myeloproliferative disorders and conditions that are associated with reactive thrombocytosis, such as iron deficiency anemia.

Table 4–2

CHARACTERISTIC FEATURES OF ESSENTIAL
THROMBOCYTHEMIA

Platelet count > 600,000/μL
Lack of Ph[1] or abl-bcr rearrangement
Normal RBC mass
Lack of iron deficiency
Absence of conditions associated with reactive thrombocytosis
Absence of or minimal bone marrow fibrosis (less than ⅓ of the biopsy
  section)
Lack of splenomegaly and leukoerythroblastic reaction

RBC = red blood cell.

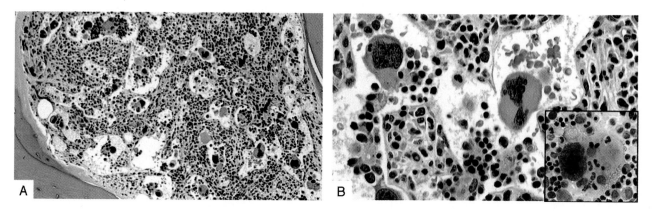

Figure 4–3. Essential thrombocythemia. Bone marrow biopsy demonstrates hypercellularity and increased numbers of megakaryocytes (*A* and *B*, low- and high-power view, respectively). Megakaryocytes appear in clusters, and some are present in the dilated sinusoids. There is no evidence of marrow fibrosis. The inset shows a megakaryocyte with emperipolesis.

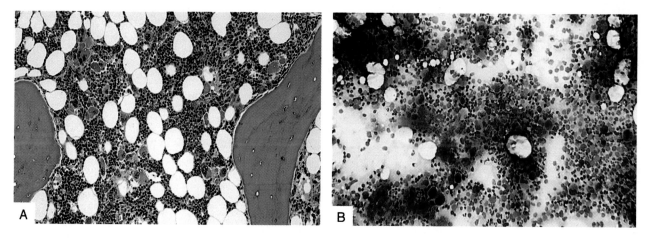

Figure 4–4. Essential thrombocythemia. Bone marrow biopsy section (*A*) and bone marrow smear (*B*) demonstrate increased megakaryocytes, some in clusters. There is no evidence of marrow fibrosis.

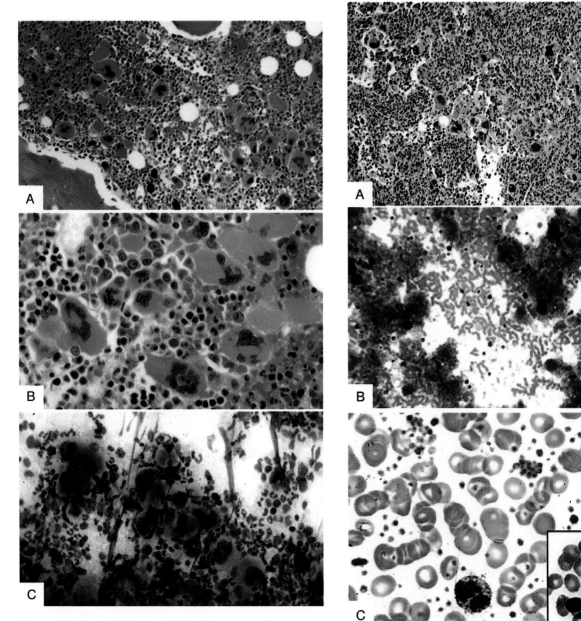

Figure 4–5. Essential thrombocythemia. Bone marrow biopsy section (*A* and *B*) and bone marrow smear (*C*) demonstrate increased megakaryocytes, some in clusters. Numerous large megakaryocytes with multilobated nuclei are present (*B*). There is no evidence of marrow fibrosis.

Figure 4–6. Essential thrombocythemia. Bone marrow biopsy section (*A*) demonstrates a hypercellular marrow with increased numbers of megakaryocytes. Bone marrow smear (*B*) shows abundant megakaryocytes and platelet aggregates, and blood smear (*C*) displays thrombocythemia. The inset depicts a blood smear with a megakaryocyte nucleus.

MYELOFIBROSIS WITH MYELOID METAPLASIA

Myelofibrosis with myeloid metaplasia (MMM) *(agnogenic myeloid metaplasia, myelofibrosis with extramedullary hematopoiesis)* is characterized by bone marrow fibrosis, extramedullary hematopoiesis and splenomegaly, leukoerythroblastic peripheral blood, and anisopoikilocytosis with the presence of teardrop-shaped erythrocytes.

Bone marrow biopsy sections show varying degrees of fibrosis and cellularity (Figures 4–7 to 4–10). In the early stages of the disease, bone marrow is hypercellular with mild to moderate fibrosis (see Figure 4–7). In the advanced stage of the disease, there is extensive fibrosis with scattered atypical megakarocytes and reduced numbers of erythroid and myeloid cells (see Figures 4–8 to 4–10). Reticulin stain shows increased amount of reticulin fibers, and trichrome stain is usually positive. Bone marrow aspiration is often unsuccessful (dry tap), but when successful demonstrates increased numbers of megakaryocytes, frequently displaying atypical features.

Blood examination reveals a leukoerythroblastic pattern with the presence of nucleated red blood cells and immature myeloid cells (see Figure 4–10). Myeloblasts are usually less than 5%, but in some cases may account for 5% to 10% of the bone marrow differential count. White blood cell (WBC) and platelet counts are usually high. Platelets may show abnormal morphology or granulation. Megakaryocytic fragments may be present.

Cytogenetic abnormalities are frequent (about 60%) with most frequent abnormalities being trisomy 1, 8, 9 and 21; monosomy 1; 7q-, 13q- and loss of Y.

Clinical Aspects

The average age of the MMM patients is about 60 years. The most frequent clinical findings are anemia and marked splenomegaly.

Differential Diagnosis

Differential diagnosis includes all other conditions that are associated with bone marrow fibrosis, such as other subtypes of CMPD, hematologic malignancies, metastatic tumors, chronic inflammations, metabolic disorders, and Paget's disease.

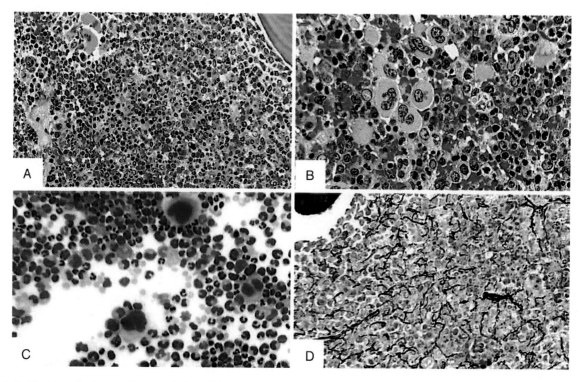

Figure 4–7. Myelofibrosis with myeloid metaplasia, cellular phase. Bone marrow biopsy section (*A* and *B*) demonstrates a hypercellular marrow with abundant megakaryocytes, some in clusters. Bone marrow smear (*C*) shows myeloid preponderance and the presence of megakaryocytes. The reticulin stain (*D*) displays moderate increase in reticulin fibers.

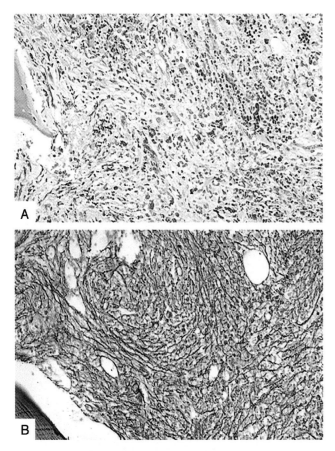

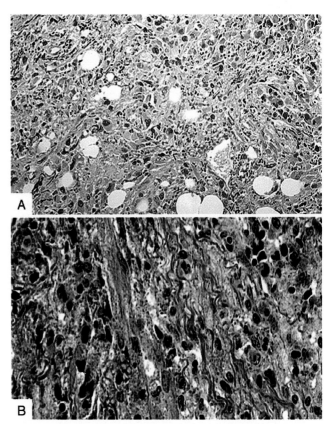

Figure 4–8. Myelofibrosis with myeloid metaplasia, advanced stage. The H & E–stained bone marrow biopsy section (A) demonstrates extensive marrow fibrosis with patchy cellular areas and scattered mega-karyocytes entrapped in the fibrotic tissue. The reticulin stain (B) shows marked increase in reticulin fibers.

Figure 4–9. Myelofibrosis with myeloid metaplasia. The H & E–stained bone marrow biopsy section (A) demonstrates myelofibrosis with numerous megakaryocytes entrapped in the fibrotic tissue. The trichrome stain (B) shows marked increase in collagen fibers (stained blue).

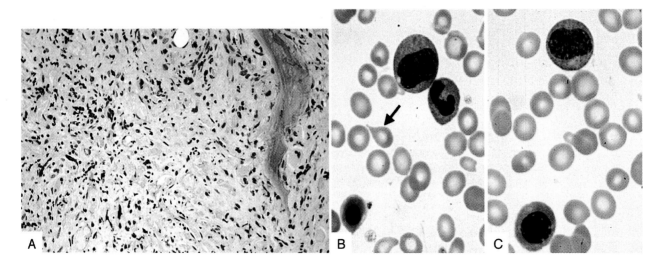

Figure 4–10. Myelofibrosis with myeloid metaplasia. Bone marrow biopsy section (A) demonstrates marked marrow fibrosis with scattered hemato-poietic cells. Peripheral blood smears (B and C) show a teardrop-shaped RBC (B, arrow), immature myeloid cells, and nucleated RBCs (leukoerythro-blastic pattern).

CHRONIC MYELOGENOUS LEUKEMIA

Chronic myelogenous *(granulocytic, myelocytic, myeloid)* leukemia (CML) is characterized by bone marrow hypercellularity and myeloid preponderance, left-shifted granulocytosis, and the presence of Ph[1] [t(9;22)(q34;q11) and the rearrangement of bcr-abl genes] (Figure 4–11). Bone marrow shows a markedly elevated myeloid:erythroid (M:E) ratio (usually >10:1) with progressive maturation of all hematopoietic lineages (Figures 4–12 and 4–13). Megakaryocytes are abundant and show marked pleomorphism ranging from small size ("dwarf" forms) to large, bizarre, multilobulated forms (Figure 4–14, see Figure 4–13). There is some degree of myeloid dysplasia, such as abnormal size and nuclear hypo- or hyperlobulation. Psuedo-Gaucher cells and/or sea-blue histiocytes are often present (see Figure 4–14). These cells are loaded with cell membrane debris, hemosiderin, and/or other phagocytic particles. Eosinophilia and basophilia are frequent findings (Figure 4–15).

Blood smears display a marked granulocytosis (commonly >50,000/μL) with a shift to the left. However, myeloblasts are usually under 5%. Eosinophilia and basophilia are common. The LAP score is low.

The transitional phase between CML and blast transformation is referred to as the *accelerated phase*. This phase is characterized by the patient's clinical deterioration evidenced by increasing degrees of anemia and thrombocytopenia, and by an increased percentage of myeloblasts (≥15%) in the bone marrow or blood (Figure 4–16; Table 4–3). Other associated findings are progressive basophilia and/or eosinophilia, increased dysplastic changes, and evidence of marrow fibrosis. The accelerated phase eventually develops into an acute leukemia *(blast transformation, blast crisis)*, which is often of myeloid origin (see Chapter 5; see Table 4–3). Approximately 15% to 30% of the transformed CMLs are of lymphoid origin or are biphenotypic. Blast transformation is often associated with additional chromosomal abnormalities, such as deletion of chromosome 17. About 70% to 80% of CML patients eventually develop blast crisis, leading to a downhill clinical course and death within 3 to 6 months.

Clinical Aspects

Approximately 20% to 30% of all adult leukemias are CML. Clinical findings are primarily related to the increased leukemic mass, the extent of splenomegaly, and the degree of abnormal granulocyte and platelet function.

Differential Diagnosis

Differential diagnosis of CML includes other subtypes of CMPD, CMML, JMML, chronic neutrophilic leukemia (see below), and leukemoid reactions. The main distinguishing features in CML are positive Ph[1]/bcl-abl and low LAP score.

Major differences between CML and leukemoid reactions are shown in Table 4–4.

Text continued on page 58

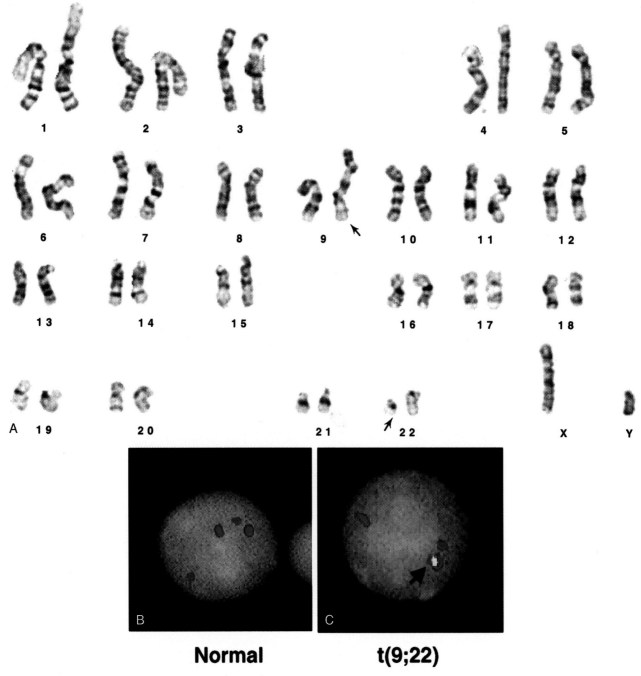

Figure 4–11. Karyotype of a male patient with chronic myelogenous leukemia (CML) demonstrating t(9;22)(q34;q11) translocation (*A*). Fluorescence in situ hybridization (FISH) analysis (*B* and *C*) with the abl (red) and bcr (green) oncogenes. Whereas two distinct green and red signals are observed in the normal nucleus (*B*), the presence of abl-bcr (yellow) fusion signal *(C, arrow)* is indicative of t(9;22). (Courtesy of Nagesh Rao, Ph.D., Department of Pathology and Laboratory Medicine, UCLA School of Medicine.)

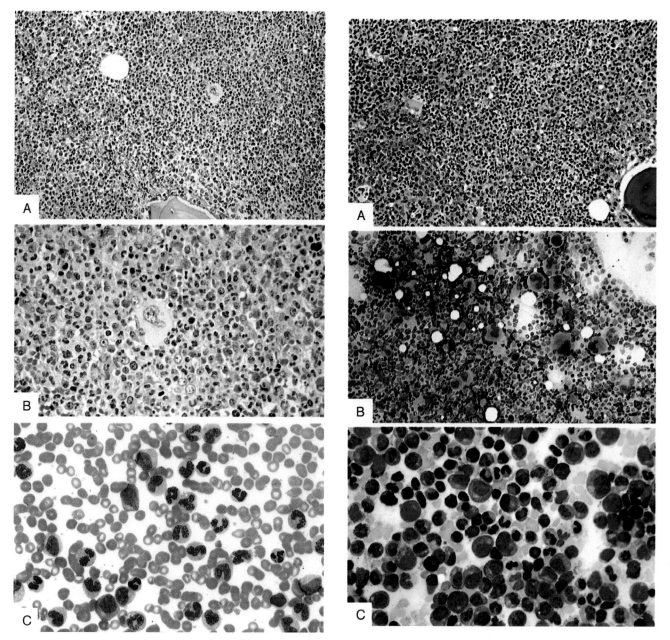

Figure 4–12. Chronic myelogenous leukemia (CML). Bone marrow biopsy section (*A* and *B*, low- and high-power views, respectively) demonstrates marked hypercellularity with elevated M : E ratio and evidence of progressive myeloid maturation. Blood smear (*C*) displays granulocytosis with a shift to the left.

Figure 4–13. Chronic myelogenous leukemia (CML). Bone marrow biopsy section (*A*) demonstrates hypercellularity with an elevated M : E ratio and evidence of progressive myeloid maturation. Bone marrow smears show a cellular marrow with numerous megakaryocytes *(B)* and marked myeloid preponderance *(C)*.

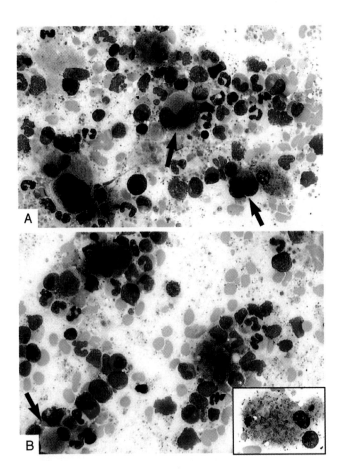

Figure 4–14. Chronic myelogenous leukemia (CML). Bone marrow smears (*A* and *B*) demonstrate micromegakaryocytes *(arrows)* and sea-blue histiocytes. The inset displays a sea-blue histiocyte containing phagocytic materials.

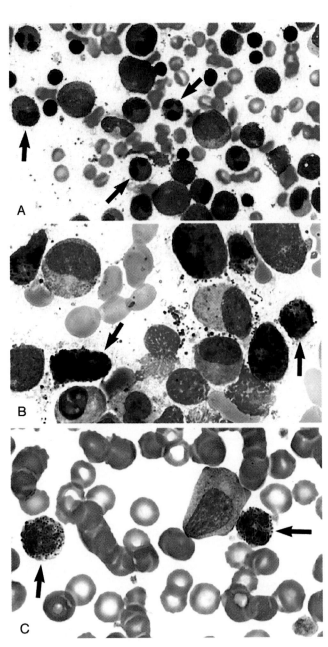

Figure 4–15. Chronic myelogenous leukemia (CML). Eosinophilia and basophilia are frequent findings in CML. Progressive basophilia has been associated with the accelerated phase and blast transformation. *A* demonstrates a bone marrow smear with eosinophilia *(arrows)*; *B* represents a bone marrow smear with basophilia, and *C* is a blood smear displaying two basophils *(arrows)* and one promyelocyte.

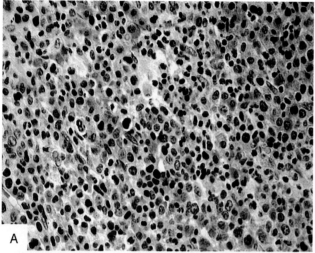

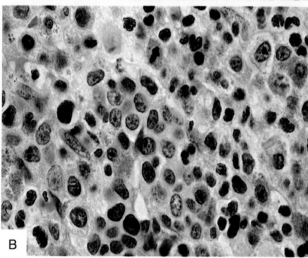

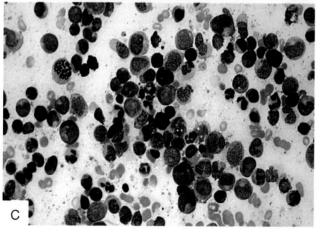

Figure 4–16. Chronic myelogenous leukemia in accelerated phase. Bone marrow biopsy section (*A* and *B*, low- and high-power views, respectively) demonstrates a marked hypercellularity with myeloid left shift and eosinophilia. Bone marrow smear (*C*) displaying myeloid left shift with increased myeloblasts.

Table 4–3

FINDINGS ASSOCIATED WITH ACCELERATED PHASE AND BLAST TRANSFORMATION IN CML

Accelerated Phase

Peripheral Blood (PB)

Progressive anemia
Marked basophilia (>20%)
Marked eosinophilia
Myeloid left shift (myeloblasts > 15%)

Bone Marrow (BM)

Myeloid left shift (myeloblasts > 15%)
Progressive basophilia and/or eosinophilia
Fibrosis

Blast Transformation

Acute myelogenous leukemia
Acute lymphoblastic leukemia
Acute biphenotypic leukemia
Other findings: Additional cytogenetic abnormalities

BM or PB blast count of >30% or >20% according to the FAB or WHO criteria, respectively.

Table 4–4

MAJOR DIFFERENCES IN LEUKEMOID REACTION AND CML

Features	Leukemoid Reaction	CML
Blood		
WBC	Often <50,000/μL	Often >50,000 μL
Early myeloid forms	Usually absent	Present
Toxic granulation	Usually present	Usually absent
Basophilia	Rare	Frequent
LAP score	Elevated	Reduced
Bone Marrow		
M:E ratio	Often <10:1	Often >10:1
Pseudo-Gaucher cells	Rare	Frequent
Basophils/mast cells	Less frequent	Frequent
Splenomegaly	Variable	Marked
Cytogenetic/DNA		
t(9;22)	Absent	Present
bcr-abl	Absent	Present

CML = chronic myelogenous leukemia; WBC = white blood cell (count); LAP = leukocyte alkaline phosphatase; M:E = myeloid:erythroid.

OTHER RELATED DISORDERS

Chronic neutrophilic leukemia, chronic eosinophilic leukemia, chronic monocytic leukemia, mast cell leukemia, and basophilic leukemia are rare conditions that, similar to the classic CPMD, represent myeloproliferation with maturation. Most of these conditions follow an aggressive clinical course and behave like an acute leukemia. Conditions associated with dysplasia and cytosis, such as CMML, atypical CML and juvenile CML, are discussed in the previous chapter.

Chronic Neutrophilic Leukemia

Chronic neutrophilic leukemia is characterized by marked neutrophilia, hepatosplenomegaly, elevated LAP, and lack of Ph[1]. Causes of leukemoid reaction, such as infections and inflammation, should be ruled out. Bone marrow is markedly hypercellular with granulocytic hyperplasia. Blood examination reveals an absolute neutrophilia (between 30,000 and 100,000/μL).

Chronic Eosinophilic Leukemia

Chronic eosinophilic leukemia *(malignant eosinophilia)* is a rare entity possessing significant overlapping features with reactive hypereosiniphilic syndromes. Marked persistent eosinophilia with the presence of immature forms, hepatosplenomegaly, and often lymphadenopathy are the main characteristic features (Figure 4–17). Cytogenetic abnormalities (such as trisomy 8), if present, are helpful to distinguish chronic eosinophilic leukemia from hypereosinophilic syndromes.

Chronic Monocytic Leukemia

Chronic monocytic leukemia is an old terminology for a rare disease characterized by massive splenomegaly and absolute monocytosis (Figure 4–18). Many of the reported cases probably fall into the more recently defined entities such as CMML and hairy cell leukemia.

Mast Cell Leukemia

Mast cell leukemia is a rare condition representing leukemic manifestation of aggressive systemic mastocytosis (Figures 4–19 and 4–20). Leukemic mast cells are atypical and pleomorphic, and often show a variable amount of cytoplasmic granules.

Basophilic Leukemia

Basophilic leukemia is an extremely rare disorder characterized by marked basophilia with a large proportion of immature forms. This disorder should be distinguished from leukemias that are associated with basophilia such as CML and certain cases of acute leukemia.

Selected References

Anderson JE, Appelbaum FR: Myelodysplasia and myeloproliferative disorders. Curr Op Hematol 4:261, 1997.

Bennett JM, Catovsky D, Daniel MT, et al: The chronic myeloid leukemias: Guidelines for distinguishing chronic granulocytic, atypical chronic myeloid, and chronic myelomonocytic leukemia. Proposal by French-American-British Cooperative Leukemia Group. Br J Haematol 87:746, 1994.

Bilgrami S, Greenberg BR: Polycythemia rubra vera. Semin Hematol 22:307, 1995.

Butturini A, Gale RP: Chronic myelogenous leukemia as a model of cancer development. Semin Oncol 22:374, 1995.

Costello R, Lafage M, Toiron Y, et al: Philadelphia chromosome-negative chronic myeloid leukemia: A report of 14 new cases. Br J Haematol 90:346, 1995.

Deininger MW, Goldman JM: Chronic myeloid leukemia. Curr Op Hematol 5:302, 1998.

Dewald GW, Wright PI: Chromosome abnormalities in the myeloproliferative disorders. Semin Oncol 22:341, 1995.

Dickstein JI, Vardiman JW: Hematopathologic findings in the myeloproliferative disorders. Semin Oncol 22:355, 1995.

Dickstein JI, Vardiman JW: Issues in pathology and diagnosis of the chronic myeloproliferative disorders and the myelodysplastic syndromes. Am J Clin Pathol 99:513, 1993.

Faderl S, Kantarjian HM, Talpaz M: Chronic myelogenous leukemia: Update on biology and treatment. Oncology 13:169, 1999.

Faderl S, Talpaz M, Estrov Z, et al: Chronic myelogenous leukemia: Biology and therapy. Ann Int Med 131:207, 1999.

Foucar K: Bone marrow pathology. Chicago, ASCP Press, 1995, p 121.

Naeim F: Pathology of Bone Marrow. Baltimore, Williams & Wilkins, 1997, p 166.

Oliver JW, Deol I, Morgan DL, et al: Chronic eosinophilic leukemia and hypereosinophilic syndromes. Proposal for classification, literature review, and report of a case with a unique chromosomal abnormality. Cancer Genet Cytogenet 107:111, 1998.

Oscier DG: Atypical chronic myeloid leukemia, a distinct clinical entity related to the myelodysplastic syndrome? Br J Haematol 92:582, 1996.

Sekhar M, Prentice HG, Popat U, et al: Idiopathic myelofibrosis in children. Br J Haematol 93:394, 1996.

Tefferi A: Pathogenetic mechanisms in chronic myeloproliferative disorders: Polycythemia vera, essential thrombocythemia, agnogenic myeloid metaplasia, and chronic myelogenous leukemia. Semin Hematol Suppl 2:3, 1999.

Tefferi A, Silverstein MN, Hoagland HC: Primary thrombocythemia. Semin Hematol 22:334, 1995.

Tefferi A: Myelofibrosis with myeloid metaplasia. N Engl J Med 342:1255, 2000.

Urbano-Ispisua A, Cervantes F, Matutes E, et al: Immunophenotypic characteristics of blast crisis of chronic myeloid leukemia: Correlations with clinico-biological features and survival. Leukemia 7:1349, 1993.

Visani G, Finelli C, Castelli U, et al: Myelofibrosis with myeloid metaplasia: Clinical and hematological parameters predicting survival in a series of 133 patients. Br J Haematol 75:4, 1990.

Wolf B, Neiman RS: Myelofibrosis with myeloid metaplasia: Pathophysiologic implications of the correlation between bone marrow changes and progression of splenomegaly. Blood 65:803, 1985.

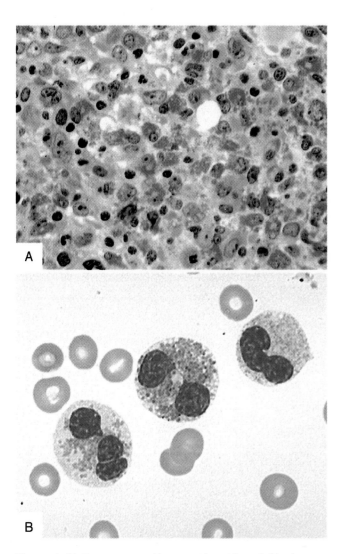

Figure 4–17. Bone marrow biopsy section (*A*) and blood smear (*B*) demonstrate eosinophilia with atypical features. There is evidence of myeloid left shift with the presence of immature eosinophils. Differential diagnosis includes hypereosinophilic syndrome and eosinophilic leukemia.

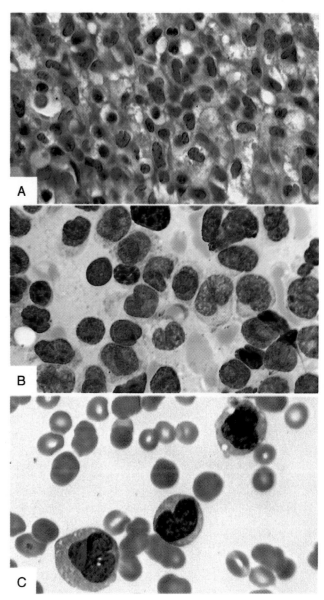

Figure 4–18. Sheets of promonocytes and monocytes are demonstrated in the bone marrow biopsy section (*A*) and marrow smear (*B*). The blood smear (*C*) shows several monocytes. This lesion was called "chronic monocytic leukemia" but probably represents a variant of chronic myelomonocytic leukemia (CMML).

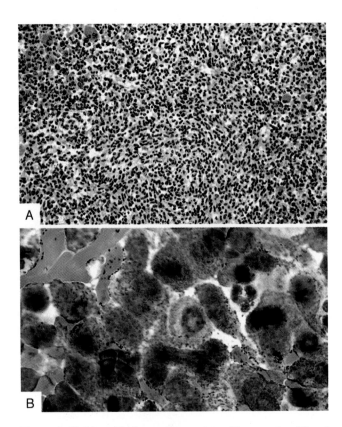

Figure 4–19. Mast cell disease. Bone marrow biopsy section (*A*) and marrow smears (*B*) demonstrate sheets of mast cells. Spindle-shaped mast cells with elongated nuclei may resemble fibroblasts (*A*).

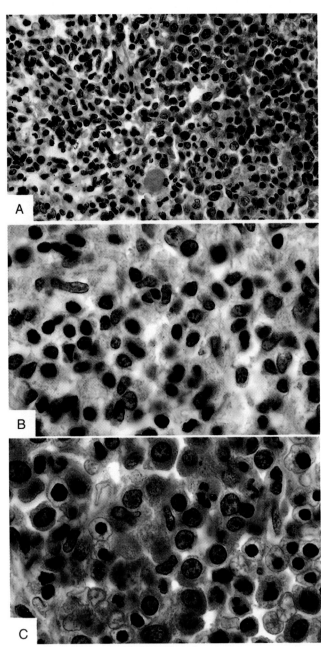

Figure 4–20. Mast cell disease. Bone marrow biopsy sections demonstrate sheets of mast cells with variable cytoplasmic granules and round or elongated nuclei (*A–C*).

CHAPTER 5

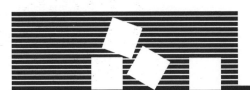

Acute Myelogenous Leukemia

Acute myelogenous leukemia (AML) represents malignancies of nonlymphoid hematopoietic precursor cells and therefore consists of a variety of cell types, including myeloblasts, promyelocytes, monoblasts, promonocytes, erythroblasts, and megakaryoblasts. AML is also referred to as *acute nonlymphoid leukemia* (ANLL), *acute granulocytic leukemia, acute myeloid leukemia, acute myeloblastic leukemia*, and *acute myelocytic leukemia*. AML, similar to the other neoplastic processes, is considered as a monoclonal disorder. Leukemogenesis appears to be a complex process. It includes at least two major steps: (1) development of a clone of abnormal precursor cells due to structural alterations or mutation of certain genes; and (2) progression to acute leukemia by further genetic changes involving one or more oncogenes and/or suppressor genes.

Myeloblasts are the predominant precursor cells in most categories of AML and are of three major morphologic types: I, II, and III (see Chapter 1) (Figure 5–1). According to the French-American-British (FAB) classification, the diagnosis of AML is established when 30% or more of the nucleated bone marrow cells and/or blood leukocytes are blasts of a nonlymphoid lineage. However, this number has been reduced to $\geq 20\%$ according to the recent classification guidelines by the World Health Organization (WHO). In addition to myeloblasts, promyelocytes (see Figure 5–10), monoblasts and promonocytes (Figure 5–2), erythroblasts and megakaryoblasts are increased in certain types of AML.

The cytochemical stains that are routinely used for the diagnosis and classification of AMLs are myeloperoxidase (MPO), Sudan black B (SBB), chloroacetate esterase (CAE), nonspecific esterases (NSE; α-naphthyl acetate or butyrate esterase), and periodic acid-Schiff (PAS) (Figure 5–3). The most frequent monoclonal antibodies (MoAbs) used for the immunophenotypic studies of AML include MoAbs against HLA-DR, CD34, CD33, CD15, CD14, CD13, CD42, CD61, CD64, CD68, and CD117 antigens, and MPO. In addition, AML cells may express certain lymphoid-associated antigens, such as CD2, CD4, CD7, CD19, CD56, and TdT (Table 5–1).

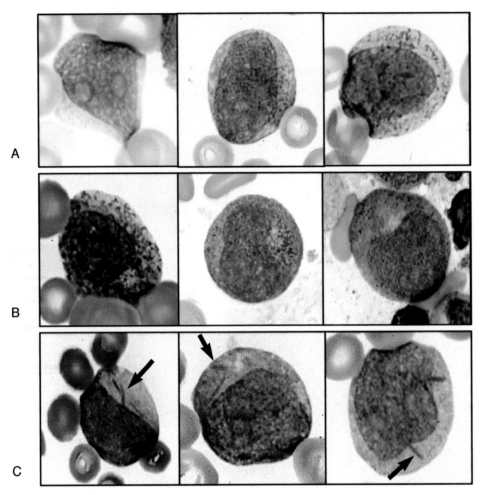

Figure 5–1. Bone marrow smears demonstrating myeloblasts type I, II, and III (*A*), promyelocytes (*B*), and Auer rods (*C*). Notice the overlapping morphologic features between myeloblasts type III (*A*, right) and promyelocytes (*B*). In general, myeloblasts are HLA-DR-positive and may express CD34, whereas promyelocytes are HLA-DR-negative and lack CD34 expression.

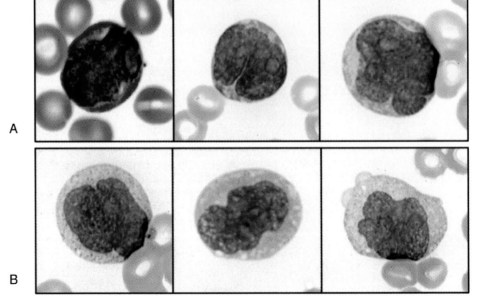

Figure 5–2. Blood smears demonstrating monoblasts (*A*) and promonocytes (*B*).

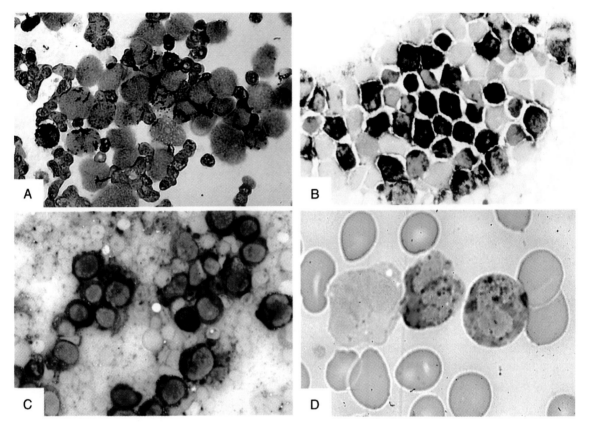

Figure 5–3. Bone marrow smears (*A*, *B*, and *C*) demonstrating positive staining for myeloperoxidase (*A*) and Sudan black B (*B*) in the granulocytic precursors, and alpha naphtyl butyrate esterase (nonspecific esterase) in monocytic precursors (*C*). A blood smear stained with chloroacetate esterase (*D*) shows positive reactions with a segmented cell and band. The negatively stained cell is a monocyte.

Table 5–1
DIFFERENTIATION-ASSOCIATED ANTIGENS FREQUENTLY
SCREENED FOR THE DIAGNOSIS AND CLASSIFICATION OF
ACUTE MYELOGENOUS LEUKEMIAS

Antigen	Primary Site of Expression
CD13	Intermediate and mature granulocytes
CD14	Monocytic lineage
CD15	Intermediate and mature granulocytes
CD33	Immature granulocytic lineage
CD34	Stem cells
CD42	Megakaryocytic lineage
CD61	Megakaryocytic lineage
CD64	Monocytic lineage
CD68	Monocytic lineage
CD117	Stem cells
HLA-DR	Blasts and monocytic lineage

CLASSIFICATION

A morphologic classification of AML was proposed by the French-American-British (FAB) Cooperative Group in 1976. The original proposal has been revised several times, and the updated version includes eight categories from M0 to M7 (Table 5–2). These categories are defined based on the morphologic and cytochemical characteristics of the leukemia cells. The recently proposed classification by the WHO is essentially similar to the FAB classification except for some revisions (Table 5–3).

Acute Myeloblastic Leukemia, Minimally Differentiated (AML-M0)

The blast cells in AML-M0 exhibit no distinctive morphologic features or cytoplasmic granules or Auer rods (Figure 5–4). Routine cytochemical stains, such as MPO, SBB, and NSE, are negative (<3% positive blast cells), but more than 20% of the blasts express myeloid-associated antigens, such as CD13 and CD33, or show the presence of MPO by immunoelectron microscopy. Blasts are often CD34+ and HLA-DR+, and may express TdT. Monosomy 5q and 7q−, and trisomy 13, have been reported in some cases of AML-M0 (see Table 5–2).

Approximately 5% of the AMLs are estimated to be M0. AML-M0 is considered an aggressive disease characterized by a low remission rate and early relapse.

Acute Myeloblastic Leukemia Without Maturation (AML-M1)

AML-M1 accounts for approximately 20% of the ANLLs and is characterized by the lack of myeloid maturation and the presence of 90% or more myeloblasts (type I and type II) in the nonerythroid component of the bone marrow (Figures 5–5 and 5–6). At least 3% of the blast cells are MPO- and/or SBB-positive. Auer rods are infrequent. AML-M1 blasts are usually positive for CD13, CD33, and HLA-DR, and may express CD34 (Figure 5–7). AML cells in a small proportion of the cases are TdT-positive.

The most frequent cytogenetic abnormalities associated with AML-M1 are t(9;22) and t(11;19).

Acute Myelogenous Leukemia With Maturation (AML-M2)

AML-M2 shows evidence of partial maturation of myeloblasts. In addition to myeloblasts, promyelocytes, myelocytes, and more mature myeloid cells are also present (Figures 5–8 and 5–9). Auer rods may be present not only in myeloblasts but in more mature cells. Myeloblasts are predominantly of types II and III, are strongly MPO- and SBB-positive, and often express HLA-DR, CD13, CD15, and CD33. Expression of CD34 and CD117 is less frequent. NSE stain is negative. Approximately 30% of ANLLs are AML-M2.

The most frequent cytogenetic abnormality associated with AML-M2 is t(8;21), observed in about 20% of the cases. These cases often show eosinophilia and CD34-positive blasts. A small proportion of the AML-M2 cases demonstrate t(6;9), often associated with bone marrow basophilia.

Acute Promyelocytic Leukemia (AML-M3)

Promyelocytes are the predominant immature cells in AML-M3. Myeloblasts are also increased, but not to the extent of promyelocytes. AML-M3 is divided into two major morphologic types: *hypergranular* and *microgranular* (hypogranular). The hypergranular variant is characterized by the presence of atypical promyelocytes heavily loaded with azurophilic granules (Figures 5–10 and 5–11). Auer rods are often present and may appear in bundles in some of the promyelocytes (faggot cells) (Figures 5–12 and 5–13). In the microgranular variant, promyelocytes contain fewer and finer (dust-like) azurophilic granules (Figures 5–14 and 5–15). The nuclei are often lobulated, folded, or convoluted, displaying a monocyte-like morphology (see Figures 5–14 and 5–15). Auer rods are often present.

The leukemia cells in AML-M3 are strongly MPO- and SBB-positive, and express CD13, CD33, CD11, and CD15 antigens, but are HLA-DR- and CD14-negative (Figure 5–16). A small proportion of cases may also demonstrate NSE reactivity.

The pathognomonic feature of AML-M3 is t(15;17), which has been observed in over 90% of the cases (Figure 5–17). This translocation puts two genes, PML and retinoic acid receptor-α (RAR-α), together with a hybrid protein product that appears to block the myeloid differentiation process. Rare cases of AML-M3 are associated with t(11;17).

Acute Myelomonocytic Leukemia (AML-M4)

In acute myelomonocytic leukemia (AMML), myeloblasts (types I, II, and III), monoblasts, and promonocytes are the predominant immature cells (Figures 5–18 and 5–19). Therefore, there is considerable pleomorphism in cell size, nuclear shape, and the amount of cytoplasm. The proportion of the monocytic component in the leukemic population ranges from more than 20% to less than 80%. Auer rods may be present but are infrequent. In addition to the bone marrow findings, patients with AML-M4 often demonstrate an absolute peripheral blood monocytosis (usually ≥5000/μL) with the presence of immature forms.

Immunophenotypic studies reveal expression of a combination of granulocytic and monocytic markers such as CD11c, CD13, CD14, CD15, CD33, CD64, CD68, and HLA-DR (Figure 5–20). The leukemia cells in some cases may also express CD2, CD4, or TdT.

The most frequent cytogenetic findings in AML-M4 are t(6;9) and 11q23 abnormalities.

Approximtely 15% to 30% of the AML-M4 cases are associated with atypical eosinophilia and abnormality of chromosome 16(q22) (Figure 5–21). The eosinophils in this subtype (AML-M4Eo) contain a mixture of eosinophilic and basophilic granules (Figures 5–22 to 5–23). The M4Eo subtype has a more favorable clinical outcome, but has a higher frequency of central nervous system (CNS) involvement.

Acute Monoblastic Leukemia (AML-M5)

Acute monoblastic *(monocytic)* leukemia (AMoL) accounts for about 10% of all ANLLs. AML-M5 is divided into two morphologic subtypes: M5a and M5b.

M5a demonstrates minimal morphologic evidence of monocytic differentiation (poorly differentiated AMoL). Monoblasts account for 80% or more of the leukemia cells. They have a variable amount of gray-blue or deep blue cytoplasm, often round or oval nuclei, and a single or a few very prominent nucleoli (Figures 5–24 and 5–25). Auer rods are usually absent.

M5b depicts partial monocytic differentiation with a mixture of monoblasts, promonocytes, and more mature monocytic cells (Figures 5–26 and 5–27). Promonocytes are characterized by abundant pale blue cytoplasm, scattered azurophilic granules, folded or lobulated nuclei, and finely dispersed chromatin (see Figure 5–2B). Nucleoli are usually not prominent. Auer rods are detected in a small proportion of the M5b subtype.

Leukemia cells are usually strongly positive for NSE and lysozyme and express all or some of the monocytic-associated markers such as CD14, CD64, CD68 (see Figures 5–24 to 5–26). They are often positive for CD4, CD11c, CD33, and HLA-DR, and may also express CD34.

Abnormalities of chromosome 11(q23) and trisomy 8 are the most frequent cytogenetic findings.

Acute Erythroid Leukemia (AML-M6)

Most acute erythroid leukemias are preceded by refractory anemia (with or without ringed sideroblasts). This early phase then evolves into refractory anemia with excess blasts (RAEB) and eventually acute erythroid leukemia. Diagnosis of AML-M6 is established based on the following bone marrow findings: (1) a reversed myeloid:erythroid (M:E) ratio (more than 50% of the marrow cells are erythroid); and (2) 30% or more of the nonerythroid marrow cells are myeloblasts (Figures 5–28 and 5–29). Erythroid lineage shows marked dysplasia, such as the presence of bi- or multinucleated erythroblasts, giant forms, and cells with nuclear fragments. Megaloblastic erythropoiesis is common. Dysplastic changes may be noted in other hematopoietic lineages. An increased number of megakaryoblasts may be present. Blood smears often show abnormal red blood cell (RBC) morphology and marked anisopoikilocytosis. The *de novo* AML-M6 accounts for about 5% of the ANLLs. The incidence is higher in the therapy-related acute leukemias.

The erythroid precursors express glycophorin A, transferrin receptor (CD71), hemoglobin, and spectrin, and may show chunk-like cytoplasmic PAS positivity. Myeloblasts are MPO- and SBB-positive and express CD13, CD33, HLA-DR, and sometimes CD34. Megakaryoblasts, if present, are defined by expressing CD42 and/or CD61.

Cytogenetic studies may demonstrate structural abnormalities in chromosomes 3, 5, and 7, or trisomy 8.

Acute pure erythroleukemia is referred to a rare condition characterized by marked erythroid preponderance and dysplasia with increased numbers of erythroblasts.

Acute Megakaryoblastic Leukemia (AML-M7)

The blast population in AML-M7 is predominantly megakaryocytic. Megakaryoblasts are pleomorphic and vary in size, amount of cytoplasm, chromatin density, and the number of nucleoli (Figure 5–30). One of the morphologic features of megakaryoblasts is cytoplasmic budding and a tendency to appear in clusters (Figure 5–31). Bone marrow fibrosis, and as a consequence unsuccessful marrow aspiration (dry tap), is one of the characteristic features of AML-M7 observed in over 70% of the cases (see Figure 5–30). Megakaryoblasts often appear in clusters trapped within the fibrotic tissue, sometimes resembling metastasis.

Megakaryoblasts and immature megakaryocytes express CD41, CD42, and CD61 (Figure 5–32), and are positive for factor VIII. They do not express MPO and SBB, but demonstrate platelet peroxidase (PPO) activity by immunoelectron microscopy and may show dot-like NSE positivity.

Blood smears often demonstrate megakaryoblasts, immature megakaryocytes, and giant platelets. Leukoerythroblastosis and anisopoikilocytosis in most instances are minimal or absent.

AML-M7 comprises about 5% of ANLLs, but is probably the most common type of AML associated with Down syndrome.

Trisomy 21 and t(1;22) have been reported in *de novo* AML-M7, and trisomy 8 and structural abnormalities of chromosomes 5 and 7 have been found in therapy-related cases.

Other Types of Acute Myelogenous Leukemia

Acute hypoplastic leukemia *(acute hypocellular leukemia)* is characterized by marked bone marrow hypocellularity and predominance of the blast cells (Figure 5–33). Blasts are usually of myeloid origin, but they may be negative for MPO or SBB stains in some cases. This leukemia is more frequently seen in elderly individuals and has a tendency to remain in the smoldering phase for some time before becoming a fulminant leukemia.

Acute myelofibrosis *(acute panmyelosis with myelofibrosis)* is characterized by pancytopenia, bone marrow hypercellularity, dysplastic hematopoiesis, increased blasts, and immature cells and fibrosis. There are overlapping features between acute myelofibrosis and acute leukemias with marrow fibrosis, particularly AML-M7 and therapy-induced and myelodysplastic syndrome (MDS)–related leukemias.

Therapy-related AML (t-AML) of patients who have received chemotherapy for other malignancies (Figure 5–34). T-AMLs are of two major categories: *topoisomerase II inhibitor–related* and *alkylating agent–related*. The former category has a shorter latency period (<3 years), is often myelomonocytic or monocytic, and is frequently associated with t(11q23). The latter demonstrates a longer latency period (4–5 years), usually passes through a myelodysplastic phase, and is often associated with del(5) and del(7).

Acute basophilic leukemia is a rare variant with evidence of basophilic differentiation in the blast and immature cells. Basophilic differentiation is detected by routine microscopic examination, ultrastructural studies, or by toluidine blue stain.

Granulocytic sarcoma (chloroma) refers to extramedullary involvement with granulocytic malignancies (CML, AML). The lesion consists of immature and mature granulocytic cells, including eosinophilic precursors, in various proportions.

Text continued on page 81

Table 5–2

ACUTE MYELOGENOUS LEUKEMIA CLASSIFICATION

Type	Key Morphology	Cytogenetics
M0	Myeloblasts >90% of the nonerythroid BM cells; no Auer rods; <3% MPO$^+$	-5, 5q-, -7, 7q-
M1	Myeloblasts >90% of the nonerythroid BM cells; rare Auer rods; >3% MPO$^+$	t(9;22)
M2	Myeloblasts >30% but <90% of the nonerythroid BM cells; frequent Auer rods	t(8;21), t(6;9)
M3	30% or more promyelocytes	t(15;17)
Subtypes: Hypergranular Microgranular		
M4	Immature monocytes comprising 20–80% of the nonerythroid BM cells	t(6;9), 5q-, 7q-
Subtype: With atypical eosinophils (M4Eo)	Eosinophils with basophilic granules	inv(16), del (16)
M5		
Subtypes: M5A; monoblastic (poorly differentiated)	Monoblasts comprising >80% of the nonerythroid BM cells	t(8;16), t(9;11), 11q-
M5B (with differentiation)	Mixture of monoblasts and more mature monocytic cells	t(8;16), t(9;11), 11q-
M6		
Subtypes: Acute pure erythroid leukemia	50% or more erythroid precursors; increased erythroblasts, marked dysplasia	
Acute erythroleukemia	50% or more erythroid precursors; 30% or more myeloblasts in the nonerythroid BM cells	5q-, 7q-, +8
M7	30% or more megakaryoblasts	+21 t(1;22)
Other Types: Acute hypocellular (hypoplastic) leukemia Acute myelofibrosis (acute panmyelosis with myelofibrosis) Therapy-related AML AML evolving from MDS and other chronic clonal hematologic disorders Acute basophilic leukemia Myeloid sarcoma (chloroma)		

BM = bone marrow; MPO = myeloperoxidase; AML = acute myelogenous leukemia; MDS = myelodysplastic syndromes.

Table 5–3

PROPOSED WHO CLASSIFICATION OF ACUTE MYELOID LEUKEMIA (AML)

AMLs with recurrent cytogenetic translocations AML with (8;21)(q22;q22), AML1(CBFα)/ETO Acute promyelocytic leukemia [AML with t(15;17)(q22; q21) and variants, PML/RARα] AML with abnormal bone marrow eosinophils inv(16)(p13q22) or t(16;16)(p13;q11), CBFβ/MYHIIX AML with 11q23 (MLL) abnormalities AMLs with multilineage dysplasia With prior myelodysplastic syndrome Without prior myelodysplastic syndrome Therapy-related AMLs Alkalating agent related Epipodophyllotoxin related Others	AMLs not otherwise categorized AML minimally differentiated AML without maturation AML with maturation Acute myelomonocytic leukemia Acute monocytic leukemia Acute erythroid leukemia Acute megakaryocytic leukemia Acute basophilic leukemia Acute panmyelosis with myelofibrosis Acute biphenotypic leukemias

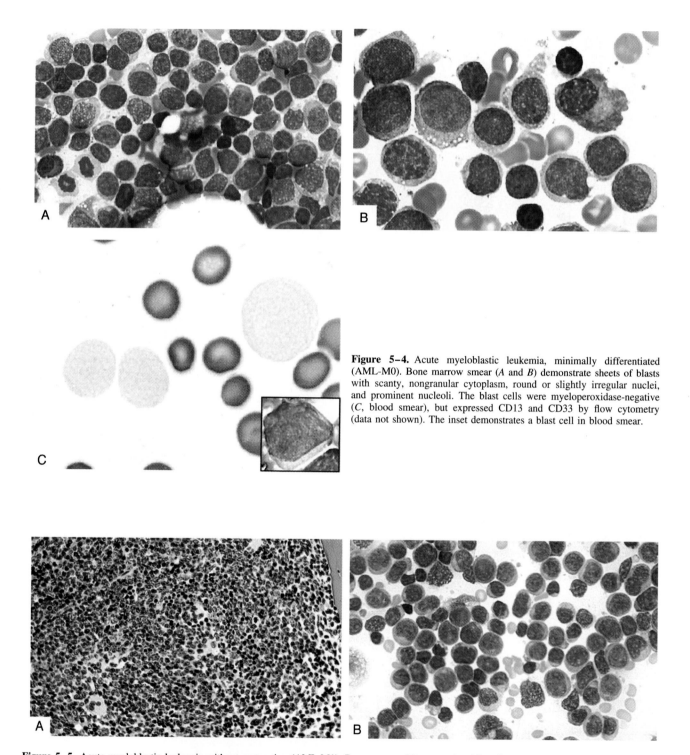

Figure 5–4. Acute myeloblastic leukemia, minimally differentiated (AML-M0). Bone marrow smear (*A* and *B*) demonstrate sheets of blasts with scanty, nongranular cytoplasm, round or slightly irregular nuclei, and prominent nucleoli. The blast cells were myeloperoxidase-negative (*C*, blood smear), but expressed CD13 and CD33 by flow cytometry (data not shown). The inset demonstrates a blast cell in blood smear.

Figure 5–5. Acute myeloblastic leukemia without maturation (AML-M1). Bone marrow biopsy section (*A*) and marrow smear (*B*) demonstrate sheets of blasts with no Auer rods and no evidence of myeloid differentiation. Morphologic features are similar to those in Figure 5–4, except that many of the blast cells in this case were positive for myeloperoxidase and Sudan black B stains (results not shown).

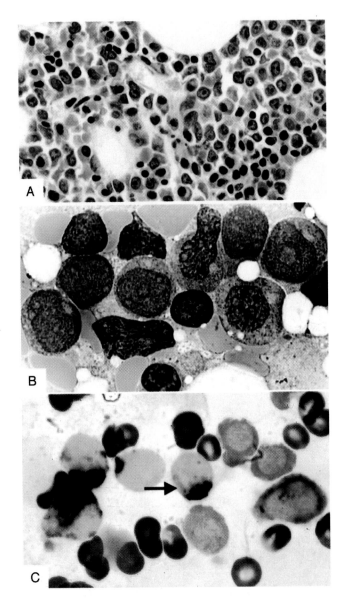

Figure 5–6. Acute myeloblastic leukemia without maturation (AML-M1). Bone marrow biopsy section (*A*) demonstrates an increased number of blast cells with scattered plasma cells. Bone marrow smear (*B*) shows several myeloblasts and a few promyelocytes. Myeloperoxidase stain displays scattered positive immature cells (*C, arrow*).

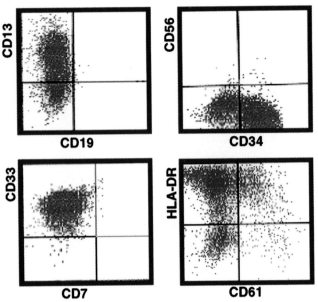

Figure 5–7. Flow cytometric results of bone marrow cells from a patient with acute myelogenous leukemia. The blast-enriched gated cells express CD13, CD33, CD34, and HLA-DR.

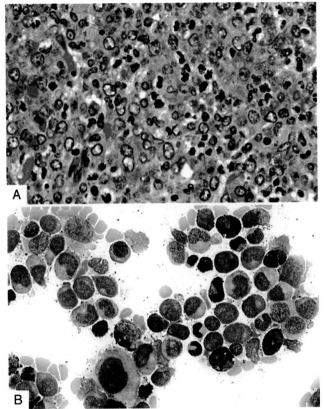

Figure 5–8. Acute myeloblastic leukemia with maturation (AML-M2). Bone marrow biopsy section (*A*) is markedly hypercellular and demonstrates a mixture of blasts and more mature cells. Bone marrow smear (*B*) shows myeloid preponderance with left shift and increased myeloblasts.

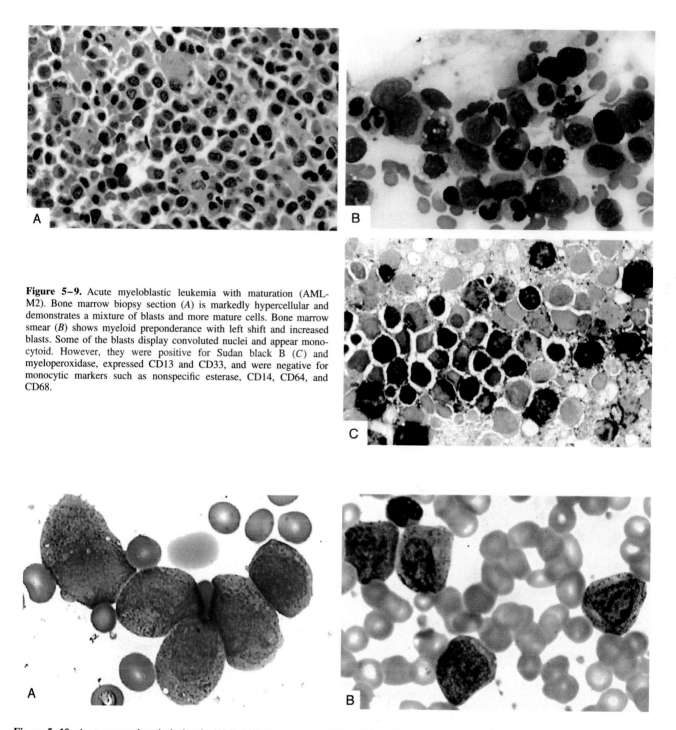

Figure 5–9. Acute myeloblastic leukemia with maturation (AML-M2). Bone marrow biopsy section (*A*) is markedly hypercellular and demonstrates a mixture of blasts and more mature cells. Bone marrow smear (*B*) shows myeloid preponderance with left shift and increased blasts. Some of the blasts display convoluted nuclei and appear mono-cytoid. However, they were positive for Sudan black B (*C*) and myeloperoxidase, expressed CD13 and CD33, and were negative for monocytic markers such as nonspecific esterase, CD14, CD64, and CD68.

Figure 5–10. Acute promyelocytic leukemia (AML-M3). Bone marrow (*A*) and blood (*B*) smears from a patient with AML-M3 demonstrate several promyelocytes with numerous coarse cytoplasmic azurophilic granules.

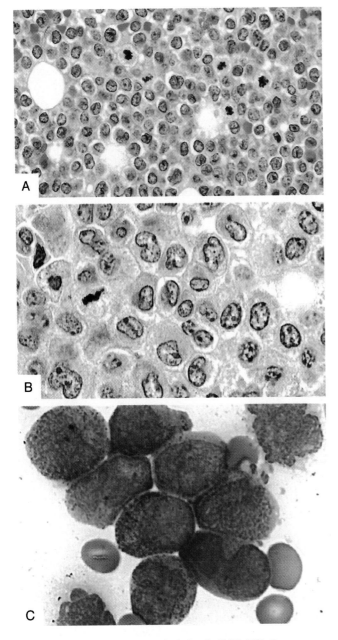

Figure 5–11. Acute promyelocytic leukemia (AML-M3). Bone marrow biopsy section (*A* and *B*) demonstrates a hypercellular marrow and sheets of immature cells with abundant granular cytoplasm and prominent nucleoi. These cells are promyelocytes as demonstrated in the bone marrow smear (*C*).

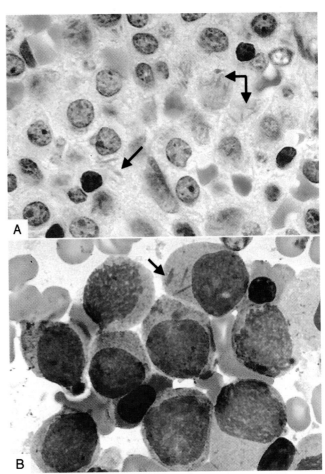

Figure 5–12. Acute promyelocytic leukemia (AML-M3). Bone marrow biopsy section (*A*) and marrow smear (*B*) demonstrate several promyelocytes containing bundles of Auer rods *(arrows)*. These cells are called faggot cells.

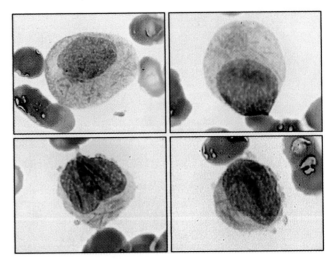

Figure 5–13. Promyelocytes with bundles of Auer rods (faggot cells).

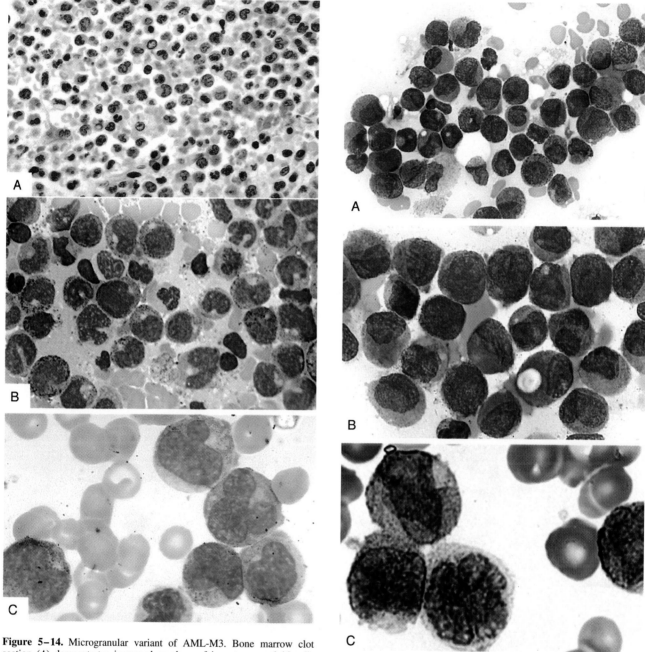

Figure 5–14. Microgranular variant of AML-M3. Bone marrow clot section (*A*) demonstrates increased numbers of immature myeloid cells with cytoplasmic granules and folded or convoluted nuclei. Bone marrow (*B*) and blood (*C*) smears show numerous promyelocytes with convoluted or folded nuclei and finely dispersed cytoplasmic granules. Scattered hypergranular promyelocytes are also present. Some of the promyelocytes with minimal or lack of granules simulate monocytes (*C*). (From Naeim F: Pathology of Bone Marrow, 2nd ed. Williams & Wilkins, 1998, with permission.)

Figure 5–15. Acute promyelocytic leukemia, microgranular variant (AML-M3v). Bone marrow (*A* and *B*) and blood (*C*) smears demonstrate numerous atypical promyelocytes with finely dispersed cytoplasmic granules and folded or convoluted nucleus. Some of these cells resemble promonocytes. Scattered heavily granulated promyelocytes are also present (*A* and *B*).

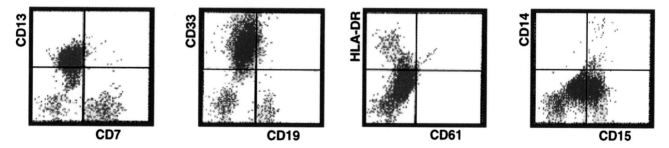

Figure 5–16. Flow cytometric analysis of a bone marrow aspirate from a patient with AML-M3. The leukemia cells express CD13, CD15, and CD33, and are negative for HLA-DR and CD14.

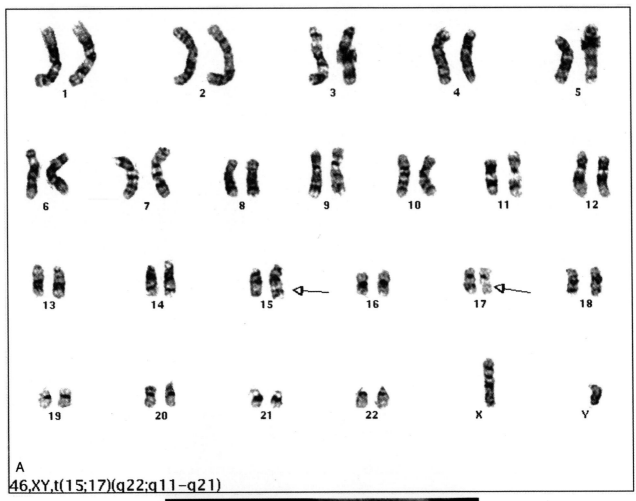

46,XY,t(15;17)(q22;q11–q21)

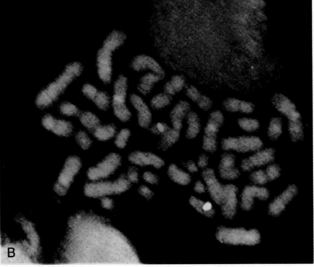

Figure 5–17. The translocation of t(15;17)(q22;q11-q21) is specifically observed in acute promyelocytic leukemia (AML-M3) (*A*). Arrows point to the regions of exchange. FISH analysis of the metaphase (*B*) showing the fusion (yellow) of the PML (green) and RARA (red) genes on chromosome 17. (Courtesy of Nagesh Rao, Ph.D., Department of Pathology and Laboratory Medicine, UCLA School of Medicine.)

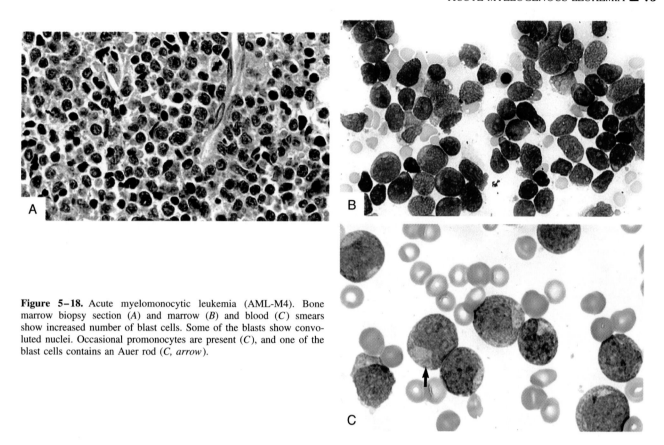

Figure 5–18. Acute myelomonocytic leukemia (AML-M4). Bone marrow biopsy section (*A*) and marrow (*B*) and blood (*C*) smears show increased number of blast cells. Some of the blasts show convoluted nuclei. Occasional promonocytes are present (*C*), and one of the blast cells contains an Auer rod (*C, arrow*).

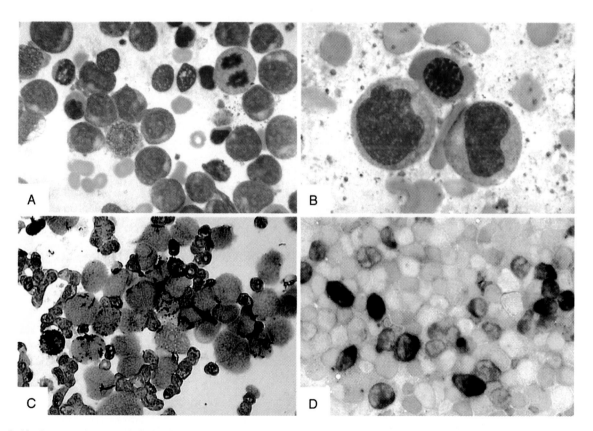

Figure 5–19. Acute myelomonocytic leukemia (AML-M4). Bone marrow smear (*A* and *B*) demonstrates increased number of blast cells. Some of the blasts show convoluted nuclei. Occasional promonocytes are present. Special cytochemical stains show a mixture of myeloperoxidase (*C*) and nonspecific esterase (*D*) positive immature cells.

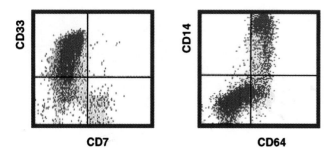

Figure 5–20. Acute myelomonocytic leukemia (AML-M4). Flow cytometric analysis of a bone marrow aspirate from a patient with AML-M4 demonstrates the expression of CD33, CD14, and CD64 by the leukemia cells.

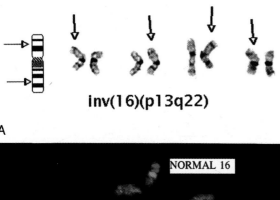

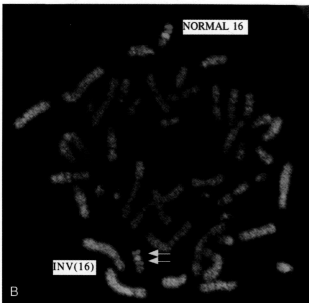

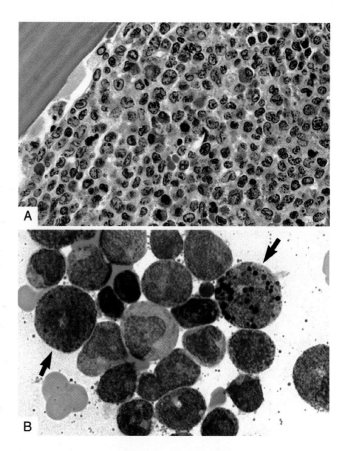

Figure 5–21. Several partial karyotypes (*A*) showing the pericentric inversion of chromosome 16 [inv(16)(p13q22)] observed in AML-4 with eosinophilia. Fluorescence in situ hybridization (FISH) analysis of the leukemia cells demonstrates the inversion sites (*B, arrows*). (Courtesy of Nagesh Rao, Ph.D., Department of Pathology and Laboratory Medicine, UCLA School of Medicine.)

Figure 5–22. Acute myelomonocytic leukemia with atypical eosinophils (AML-M4 Eo). Bone marrow biopsy section (*A*) and marrow smear (*B*) demonstrate numerous immature myelomonocytic cells and increased number of eosinophils. Some of the eosinophils contain basophilic granules (*B*).

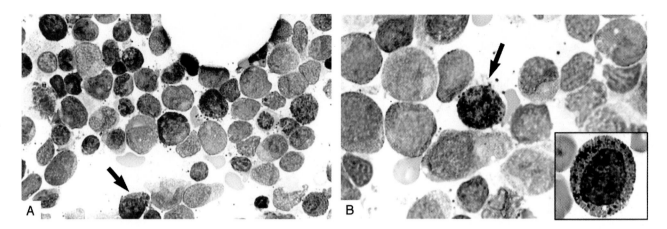

Figure 5–23. Acute myelomonocytic leukemia with atypical eosinophils (AML-M4 Eo). Bone marrow smears demonstrate numerous blasts, promonocytes, and increased number of eosinophils (*A* and *B*). Some of the eosinophils contain basophilic granules *(arrows)*. An eosinophilic myelocyte with basophilic granules is demonstrated in the inset.

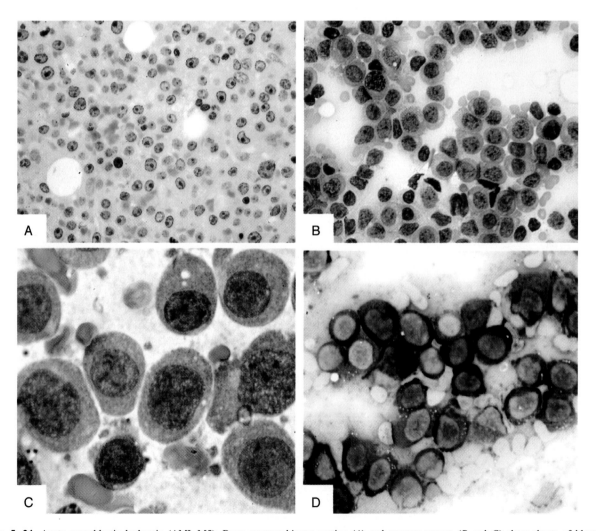

Figure 5–24. Acute monoblastic leukemia (AML-M5). Bone marrow biopsy section (*A*) and marrow smears (*B* and *C*) show sheets of blast cells with abundant cytoplasm, round nuclei, and prominent nucleoli with minimal monocytic differentiation (AML-M5a). Nonspecific esterase stain of the bone marrow smear demonstrates numerous positive cells (*D*).

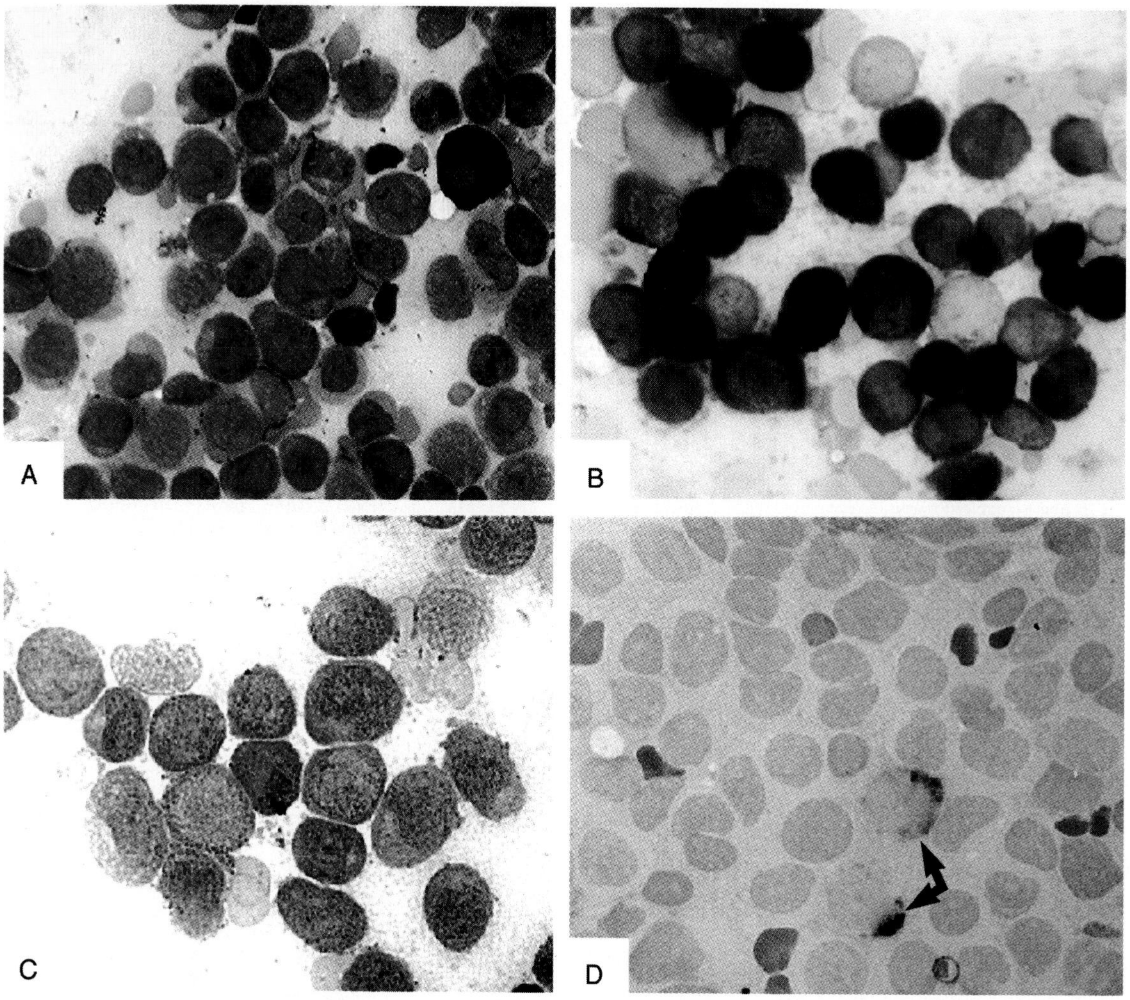

Figure 5–25. Acute monoblastic leukemia (AML-M5). Bone marrow smear (*A*) demonstrates numerous blasts with minimal monocytic differentiation (AML-M5a). Special cytochemical stains on the bone marrow smears show numerous nonspecific esterase–positive cells (*B*), several cells with coarse PAS-positive cytoplasmic granules (*C*), and occasional myeloperoxidase-positive cells (*D*).

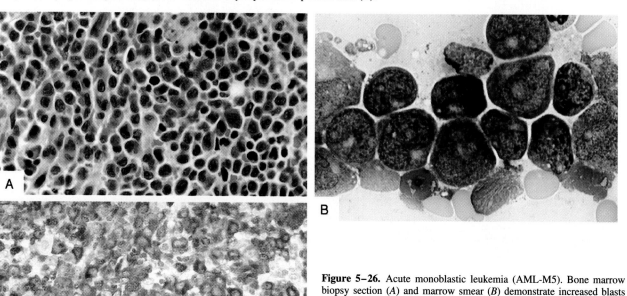

Figure 5–26. Acute monoblastic leukemia (AML-M5). Bone marrow biopsy section (*A*) and marrow smear (*B*) demonstrate increased blasts and immature monocytic cells, many with nuclear folding or convolution (AML-M5b). Immunohistochemical stain on bone marrow biopsy section shows sheets of CD68-positive cells (*C*).

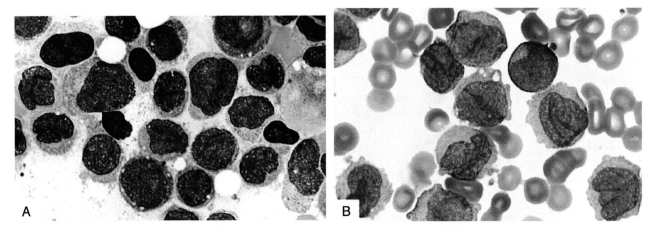

Figure 5–27. Acute monoblastic leukemia (AML-M5). Bone marrow smear (*A*) demonstrates increased blasts with nuclear folding or convolution (AML-M5b). Blood smear (*B*) shows several promonocytes and one blast cell. In AML-M4 and -M5, the monocytic component in the peripheral blood often appears more mature than the bone marrow.

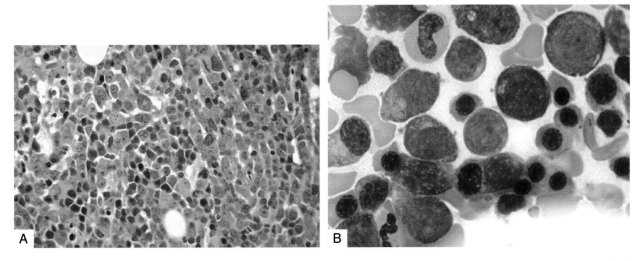

Figure 5–28. Erythroleukemia (AML-M6). Bone marrow biopsy section (*A*) demonstrates hypercellularity with marked increase in blast cells. Bone marrow smear (*B*) shows a mixture of myeloblasts and early erythroid precursors.

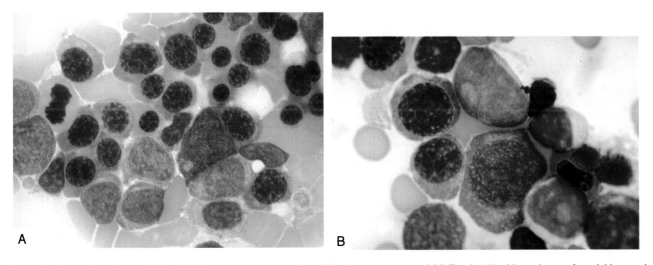

Figure 5–29. Erythroleukemia (AML-M6). Bone marrow smears (*A* and *B*) demonstrate reversed M:E ratio (*A*) with a mixture of myeloblasts and early eythroid precursors (*A* and *B*).

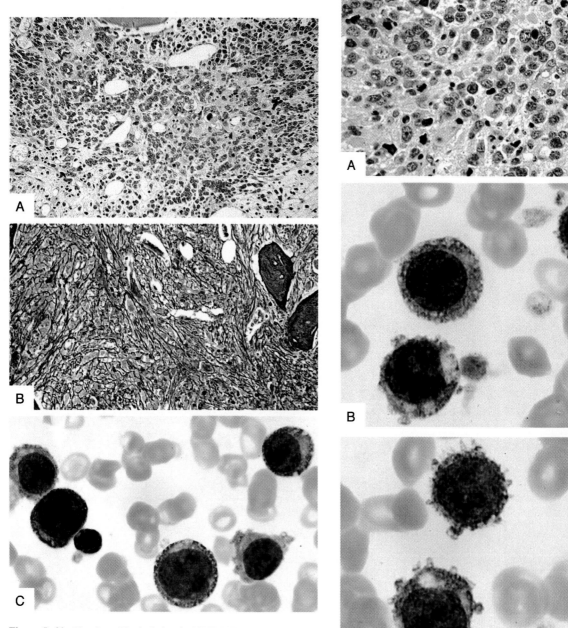

Figure 5–30. Megakaryoblastic leukemia (AML-M7). Bone marrow biopsy sections demonstrate aggregates of blast cells (A) and increased reticulin fibers (B, reticulin stain). Blood smear (C) shows several blasts in different sizes and with variable amounts of cytoplasm.

Figure 5–31. Megakaryoblastic leukemia (AML-M7). Bone marrow biopsy sections demonstrate aggregates of blast cells (A), and blood smears (B and C) show several blasts, some with cytoplasmic budding.

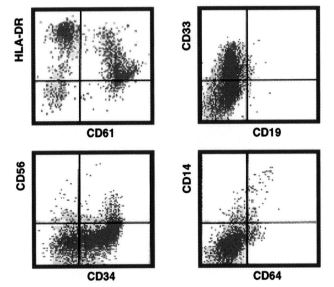

Figure 5–32. Megakaryoblastic leukemia (AML-M7). Flow cytometric analysis demonstrates a population of cells expressing CD33, CD34, CD61, and HLA-DR.

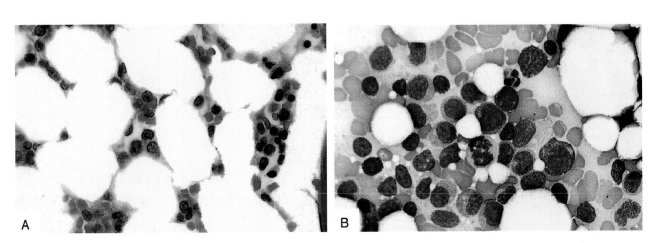

Figure 5–33. Hypocellular AML. Bone marrow biopsy section (*A*) demonstrates a hypocellular marrow, and bone marrow smear (*B*) shows increased numbers of myeloblasts.

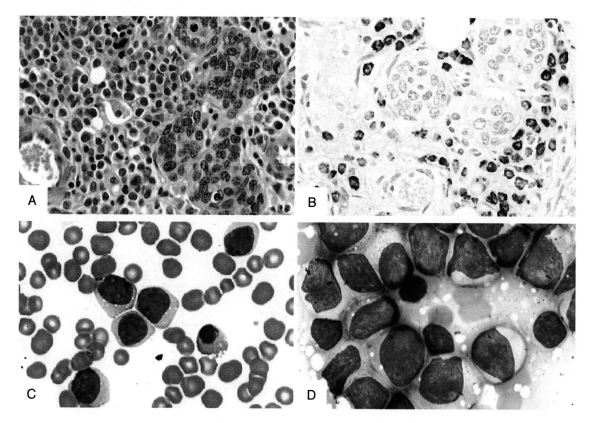

Figure 5–34. Therapy-related AML in a patient with a history of chemotherapy for adenocarcinoma of breast. Bone marrow biopsy *(A)* demonstrates sheets of blast cells mixed with several clusters of metastatic carcinoma. The blast cells are myeloperoxidase-positive *(B)*. Blood smear *(C)* and biopsy touch preparation *(D)* show numerous myeloblasts.

Table 5–4
MAJOR DIFFERENCES BETWEEN MICROGRANULAR AML-M3
AND AML-M5

Features	AML-M3	AMI-M5
Azurophilic granules	More frequent	Less frequent
MPO/SBB	Often strong	Often weak
NSE	Often negative	Often positive
Auer rods	Frequent	Rare
CD4	Negative	Often positive
CD14	Negative	Positive
HLA-DR	Negative	Positive
Cytogenetic	t(15;17)	Often 11q23 abnormalities

AML = acute myelogenous leukemia; MPO = myeloperoxidase; SBB = Sudan black B; NSE = nonspecific esterase.

CLINICAL ASPECTS

Acute myelogenous leukemias comprise about 80% of acute leukemias in adults and 15% to 20% of the childhood acute leukemias. Clinical symptoms are essentially related to the cytopenias and extramedullary involvements. Hepatomegaly and splenomegaly are observed in about 30% of the cases. Involvement of the other tissues/organs, such as skin, gastrointestinal tract, respiratory system, and urogenital tracts, is more prominent in AML-4 and AML-5. Lymphadenopathy is infrequent. Bleeding complications are more characteristic of AML-M3, but are also seen in some cases of AML-M5 and in patients with severe thrombocytopenia.

Increased blasts in blood, thrombocytopenia, and absence of Auer rods are signs of poor prognosis. Also, chromosomal deletions, multiple chromosomal abnormalities, and hyperdiploidy indicate an aggressive clinical course.

DIFFERENTIAL DIAGNOSIS

Acute myelogenous leukemia is distinguished from MDS variants, such as CMML and RAEB, on the basis of the blast counts in the bone marrow or blood samples. The differential diagnosis of M0, M1, M5A, and M7 from ALL (L1 and L2) is sometimes difficult and may require additional laboratory work, such as special stains, and immunophenotypic, cytogenetic, and molecular studies. The microgranular variant of AML-M3 is distinguished from AML-M4 and -M5 by strong positive staining for MPO and SBB, lack of expression of HLA-DR and CD14, and the presence of t(15;17) (Table 5–4). A subtype of AML-M1 shares similar morphologic and immunophenotypic features with microgranular variant of AML-M, but lacks t(15–17).

Differential diagnosis of AML in children with Down syndrome includes transient myeloproliferative disorder (see Chapter 12). This condition is usually observed within the first month of birth and disappears spontaneously after several weeks.

Selected References

Adriansen HJ, Boekhorst PAW, Hagemeijer AM, et al: Acute myeloid leukemia M4 with bone marrow eosinophilia (M4Eo) and inv (16)(p13;q22) exhibits a specific immunophenotype with CD2 expression. Blood 81:3043, 1993.

Atkinson J, Hrisinko MA, Weil SC: Erythroleukemia: A review of 15 cases meeting 1985 FAB criteria and survey of the literature. Blood Rev 6:204, 1993.

Bennett JM, Catovsky D, Daniel MT, et al: Criteria for the diagnosis of acute leukemia of megakaryocytic lineage (M7). A report of the French-American-British Cooperative Group. Ann Intern Med 103:460, 1985.

Bennett JM, Catovsky D, Daniel M-T, et al: Proposal for the recognition of minimally differentiated acute myeloid leukemia (AML-M0). Br J Haematol 78:325, 1991.

Bennett JM, Catovsky D, Daniel MT, et al: Proposals for the classification of the acute leukemias. Br J Haematol 33:451, 1976.

Bennett JM, Catovsky D, Daniel MT, et al: Proposed revised criteria for the classification of acute myeloid leukemia. A report of the French-American-British Cooperative Group. Ann Intern Med 103:620, 1985.

Cason JD, Trujillo JM, Estey EH, et al: Peripheral acute leukemia: High peripheral but low-marrow blast count. Blood 74:1758, 1989.

Cohen PL, Hoyer JD, Kurtin PL, et al: Acute myelogenous leukemia with minimal differentiation. A muliple parameter study. Am J Clin Pathol 109:32, 1998.

Cripe LD, Hromas R: Malignant disorders of megakaryocytes. Sem Hematol 35:200, 1998.

Duchayne E, Demur C, Rubie H, et al: Diagnosis of acute basophilic leukemia. Leuk Lymph 32:269, 1999.

Gassmann W, Löffler H: Acute megakaryoblastic leukemia. Leuk Lymph 18(Suppl 1):69, 1995.

Grignani F, Fagioli M, Alcalay M, et al: Acute promyelocytic leukemia: From genetics to treatment. Blood 83:10, 1994.

Harris NL, Jaffe ES, Diebold J, et al: The World Health Organization classification of hematological malignancies. Report of the Clinical Advisory Committee Meeting. Airlie House, Virginia, November 1997. Mod Pathol 13:193, 2000.

Lorand-Metze I, Vassallo J, Aoki RY, et al: Acute megakaryoblastic leukemia: Importance of bone marrow biopsy in diagnosis. Leuk Lymphoma 7:75, 1991.

Naeim F: Pathology of Bone Marrow. Baltimore, Williams & Wilkins, 1997, p 194.

O'Connor SJ, Evans PA, Morgan GJ: Diagnostic approaches to acute promyelocytic leukaemia. Leuk Lymph 33:53, 1999.

Olopade OI, Thangavelu M, Larson RA: Clinical, morphologic, and cytogenetic characteristics of 26 patients with acute erythroleukemia. Blood 80:2873, 1992.

Peterson LC, Parkin JL, Arthur DC, et al: Acute basophilic leukemia. A clinical, morphologic and cytogenetic study of eight cases. Am J Clin Pathol 96:160, 1991.

Sempere A, Jarque I, Guinot M, et al: Acute myeloblastic leukemia with minimal myeloid differentiation (FAB AML-M0): A study of eleven cases. Leuk Lymphoma 12:103, 1993.

Vardiman JM, Head D: Society for Hematopathology: The myelodysplastic syndrome (MDS) and related disorders. Mod Pathol 12:101, 1999.

Venditti A, Del Poeta G, Buccisano F, et al: Minimally differentiated acute myeloid leukemia (AML-M0): Comparison of 25 cases with other French-American-British subtypes. Blood 89:621, 1997.

Warrell RPJ, De The H, Wang ZY, et al: Acute promyelocytic leukemia. N Engl J Med 329:117, 1993.

Yumura-Yagi K, Hara J, Tawa A, et al: Phenotypic characteristics of acute megakaryocytic leukemia and transient abnormal myelopoiesis. Leuk Lymphoma 13:393, 1994.

CHAPTER 6

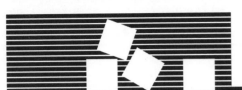

Acute Lymphoblastic Leukemia

Acute lymphoblastic *(lymphocytic, lymphoid, lymphatic)* leukemia (ALL) is a malignancy resulting from clonal proliferation of abnormal lymphoid precursors. The process of the development of ALL, similar to acute myelogenous leukemia (AML), is often associated with chromosomal aberrations involving oncogenes and suppressor genes.

Bone marrow is usually extensively infiltrated by lymphoblasts causing a marked reduction in the normal hematopoietic components and consequently pancytopenia. The pattern of bone marrow infiltration is often diffuse or interstitial. Focal or patchy involvement is infrequent. ALL infiltration is sometimes associated with marrow fibrosis or may display areas of necrosis. Lymphoblasts may appear monomorphic or pleomorphic. They have scanty to moderate amounts of cytoplasm, usually lack cytoplasmic granules, display fine nuclear chromatin, and contain one or more nucleoli.

Periodic acid-Schiff (PAS) is the only cytochemical stain that is routinely used for the diagnosis of ALL. However, this stain is not specific for lymphoid malignancies, and a similar pattern of PAS staining has been observed in dysplastic erythroid and monocytic precursors. Lymphoblasts often demonstrate coarse PAS-positive cytoplasmic granules (Figure 6–1). They are myeloperoxidase (MPO)-negative, but occasionally depict a few Sudan black B (SBB)-positive cytoplasmic granules or display focal (dot-like) cytoplasmic nonspecific esterase (NSE) positivity. The most frequent monoclonal antibodies (MoAbs) used for the immunophenotypic studies of ALL include MoAbs against CD2, CD3, CD5, CD7, CD10, CD19, CD20, CD22, CD34, CD38, HLA-DR, and TdT. In addition, in some cases, ALL leukemia cells may express certain myeloid-associated markers, such as CD15, CD13, CD14, and CD33.

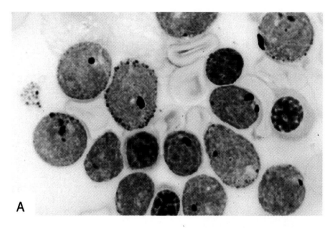

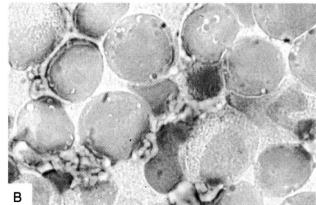

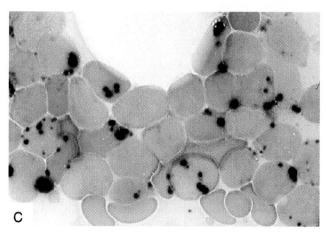

Figure 6–1. Special cytochemical stains on bone marrow smears of patients with acute lymphoblastic leukemia (ALL). *A*, Periodic acid-Schiff (PAS) stain demonstrates coarse PAS-positive cytoplasmic granules in several blast cells. *B*, Oil red O stain shows positive cytoplasmic vacuoles (round pale red stains) in the leukemia cells in Burkitt's type ALL. *C*, Nonspecific esterase stain displays dot-like cytoplasmic positivity in the blast cells.

CLASSIFICATION

Morphologic Classification

According to the French-American-British (FAB) classification, lymphoblasts are of three morphologic types: L1, L2, and L3 (Table 6–1; Figures 6–2 and 6–3). The L1 lymphoblasts are small and monomorphic with scanty blue cytoplasm; round, oval, or slightly irregular nucleus; finely dispersed chromatin; and small and inconspicuous nucleoli (Figure 6–4; see Figures 6–2 and 6–3). The L2 lymphoblasts are larger and demonstrate significant pleomorphism. They have a variable amount of cytoplasm, nuclear irregularity is more dramatic, and nucleoli are more prominent than the L1 blasts (Figure 6–5; see Figures 6–2 and 6–3). The L3 lymphoblasts are monomorphic; and depict a deep blue, often vacuolated cytoplasm; round or oval nucleus; finely dispersed chromatin; and one or more prominent nucleoli (Figures 6–6 to 6–8; see Figures 6–2 and 6–3). The L3 cells share morphologic

and immunophenotypic featutes of the neoplastic cells in Burkitt's lymphoma. They express B cell–associated antigens and surface membrane immunoglobulin. The cytoplasmic vacuoles often contain neutral fat and stain positively with oil red O stain. The WHO classification designates two major categories for ALL, L1/L2 and L3 (Burkitt's type). The L1 and L2 morphologies do not predict immunophenotype, genetic abnormalities or clinical behavior, and therefore are included in one category.

Morphologic Variants

ALL, hand-mirror cell variant, is a morphologic variant in which a significant proportion (usually ≥40%) of the leukemia cells demonstrate a cytoplasmic tail (Figure 6–9*A*). Although the majority of the reported cases of hand-mirror leukemia are ALL (usually L2 type), this morphologic variant has been also observed in AMLs. Hand-mirror morphology does not carry any clinical significance.

ALL with cytoplasmic granules (granular ALL) is usually of ALL-L2 type and accounts for about 5% of the ALLs. Blast cells contain cytoplasmic azurophilic granules and may express natural killer (NK)–associated antigens (see below) (Figures 6–9B and 6–10). This variant has been associated with a relatively poor prognosis.

ALL with eosinophilia is a rare entity usually observed in older patients and has been reported in association with t(5;14) (Figures 6–9C and D).

Immunologic Classification

There are two major immunophenotypic classes of ALL: B-lineage and T-lineage (Table 6–2).

B-Lineage ALL

This class of leukemia comprises over 80% of ALLs. It consists of four subtypes: early precursor, precursor, pre-B, and B. The most prominent immunophenotypic features of the B-lineage ALLs are demonstrated in Table 6–2.

Early precursor B-ALL accounts for about 5% of the B-lineage ALLs. The lymphoblasts are positive for TdT, HLA-DR, and CD34, and may express CD19. The most frequent cytogenetic abnormalities associated with this category are t(4;11) and t(9;22).

Precursor B-ALL (common ALL) is the most common ALL variant, accounting for over 75% of the cases. The lymphoblasts are positive for CD10 (common acute lymphoblastic leukemia antigen, CALLA), CD19, HLA-DR, and TdT, and may express CD34 and CD20 (Figure 6–11). Cytogenetic abnormalities include 6q-, 12q-, and t(5;14). ALL with t(5;14) is often associated with eosinophilia.

Pre–B-ALL is defined as a B-lineage leukemia with the presence of cytoplasmic Igμ heavy chain (cμ). The lymphoblasts also express HLA-DR, CD19, and CD20. The most frequent cytogenetic abnormalities include t(1; 19) and t(9;22).

B-ALL is the most differentiated subtype characterized by the expression of surface Ig (Figure 6–12). The lymphoblasts are also positive for HLA-DR, CD19, and CD20, and may express CD10. B-ALL corresponds to the L3 (Burkitt's type) morphology and is associated with t(8;14), t(2;8), and t(8;22) translocations, all involving 8q24.

T-Lineage ALL

Blast cells in the majority of T-lineage ALLs express prethymic or early thymic differentiation antigens, such as CD2, cytoplasmic CD3, CD5, CD7, and TdT (Figure 6–13). CD3 is not expressed on the surface of the tumor cells in the majority of cases. Blasts in approximately 30% of the T-lineage leukemias may demonstrate end-stage differentiation antigens, such as CD4 and/or CD8. T-lineage ALLs are divided into four types based on their immunophenotypic features: *early precursor, immature thymocyte, intermediate thymocyte,* and *mature thymocyte* (see Table 6–2). A rare T-ALL subtype has been reported characterized by the expression of CD16, CD56, and CD57 (NK-phenotype) on the lymphoblasts. Blast cells are also CD2- and CD8-positive and may show cytoplasmic azurophilic granules. CD3 is positive in some cases (NK-like T-ALL) and negative in others (true NK-ALL).

Cytogenetic abnormalities in T-ALLs frequently involve chromosomes 1, 7, 8, and 11, and they are mostly translocations, such as t(1;7), t(1;14), t(8;14), and t(11;14).

Text continued on page 90

Table 6–1
FRENCH-AMERICAN-BRITISH CLASSIFICATION OF ACUTE LYMPHOBLASTIC LEUKEMIA*

Features	L1	L2	L3 (Burkitt's type)
Cell size	Predominantly small	Large; polymorphic	Large; monomorphic
Cytoplasm	Scanty	Abundant	Moderate, deep blue, often vacuolated
Nucleus	Monomorphic, often regular	Polymorphic, often irregular	Monomorphic, regular
Immunophenotype	B or T	B or T	B, surface Ig-positive
Cytochemical stains	Often PAS-positive	Often PAS-positive	Often oil red O–positive

*Recent World Health Organization (WHO) proposal combines L1 and L2 subtypes together in one category and suggests only two major ALL subtypes: L1/L2 and L3.
PAS = periodic acid-Schiff; ALL = acute lymphoblastic leukemia.

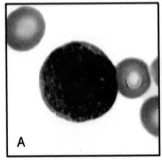 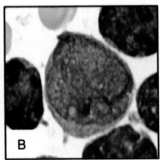 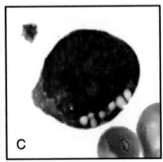

Figure 6–2. Acute lymphoblastic leukemia. L1 (*A*), L2 (*B*), and L3 (*C*) lymphoblasts.

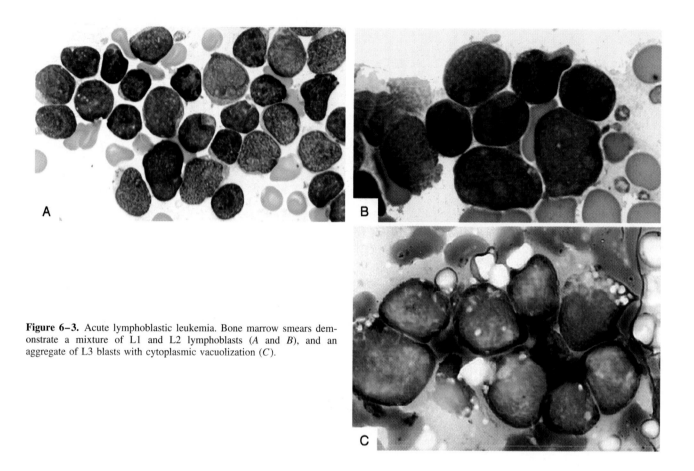

Figure 6–3. Acute lymphoblastic leukemia. Bone marrow smears demonstrate a mixture of L1 and L2 lymphoblasts (*A* and *B*), and an aggregate of L3 blasts with cytoplasmic vacuolization (*C*).

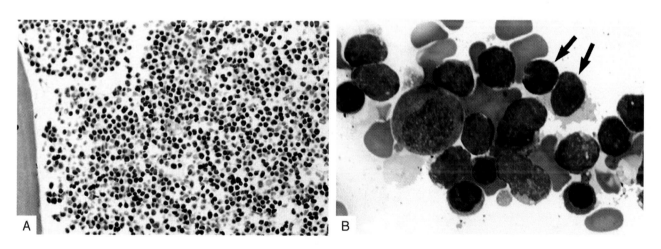

Figure 6–4. Acute lymphoblastic leukemia (ALL-L1). Bone marrow biopsy section (*A*) and marrow smear (*B*) demonstrate monomorphous lymphoblasts with scanty cytoplasm, round or slightly irregular nuclei, and inconspicuous nuclei (*arrows*).

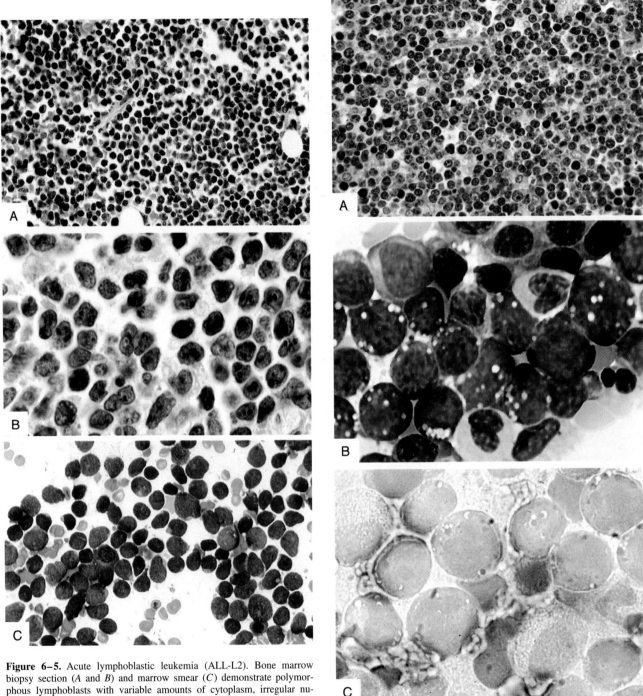

Figure 6–5. Acute lymphoblastic leukemia (ALL-L2). Bone marrow biopsy section (*A* and *B*) and marrow smear (*C*) demonstrate polymorphous lymphoblasts with variable amounts of cytoplasm, irregular nuclei, and some with prominent nucleoli.

Figure 6–6. Acute lymphoblastic leukemia (ALL-L3). Bone marrow biopsy section (*A*) and marrow smear (*B*) demonstrate monomorphic lymphoblasts with vacuolated cytoplasm and round or slightly irregular nuclei. Several blasts show prominent nucleoli. Oil red O stain of the marrow smears shows several positive cells (*C*).

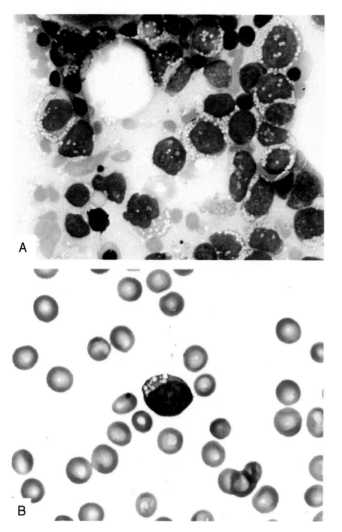

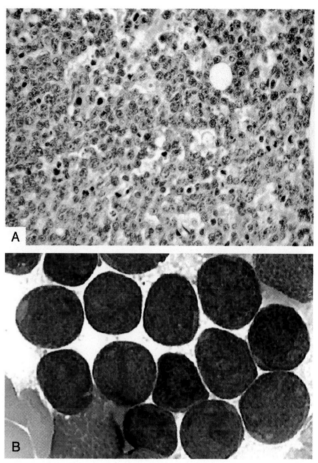

Figure 6–7. Acute lymphoblastic leukemia (ALL-L3). Bone marrow (*A*) and blood (*B*) smears demonstrate lymphoblasts with vacuolated cytoplasm. (*A*, from Naeim F: Pathology of Bone Marrow, 2nd ed. Baltimore, Williams & Wilkins, 1998, with permission.)

Figure 6–8. Acute lymphoblastic leukemia (ALL-L3). Bone marrow biopsy section (*A*) and marrow smear (*B*) demonstrate monomorphic lymphoblasts with scanty cytoplasm, round or slightly irregular nuclei, and prominent nucleoli. Note absence of cytoplasmic vacuolization. Flow cytometric studies demonstrated expression of surface kappa light chain by the blast cells and negative TdT (results not shown).

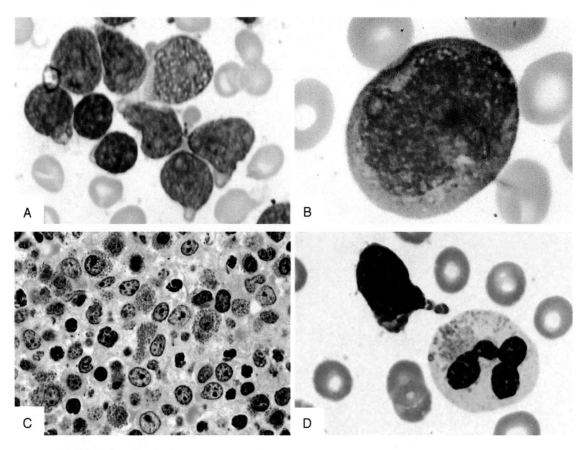

Figure 6–9. Acute lymphoblastic leukemia, morphologic variants. *A,* Bone marrow smear demonstrates ALL with hand-mirror–type blast cells. *B,* A lymphoblast with cytoplasmic azurophilic granules. *C* and *D,* ALL with eosinophilia; bone marrow biopsy section displays a mixture of lymphoblasts with eosinophils (*C*), and blood smear shows a lymphoblast and an atypical eosinophil (*D*).

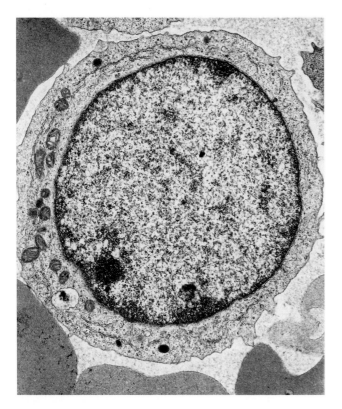

Figure 6–10. Electron microscopic image of a lymphoblast with scattered lysosomal granules from a patient with granular ALL.

Table 6–2

IMMUNOPHENOTYPIC CLASSIFICATION
OF ACUTE LYMPHOBLASTIC LEUKEMIA

Cell Type	Classification	Expression
B-Lineage	Early precursor	HLA-DR, TdT, CD19, CD34
	Precursor (common)	HLA-DR, TdT, CD19, CD34($\pm$), CD10, CD20($\pm$)
	Pre-B	HLA-DR, TdT ($\pm$), CD10, CD19, CD20, cytoplasmic μ
	B	HLA-DR, CD19, CD10($\pm$), CD20, surface membrane Ig
T-Lineage	Early precursor	CD7, TdT, CD34
	Immature thymocyte	CD7, TdT, CD38, cytoplasmic CD3, CD5, CD2, CD34($\pm$)
	Intermediate thymocyte	CD7, TdT, CD5, CD38, CD2, CD3, CD4, CD8
	Mature thymocyte	CD7, CD2, CD5, CD38, CD3, CD4 or CD8, TdT($\pm$)

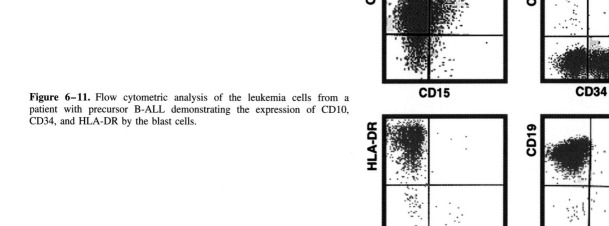

Figure 6–11. Flow cytometric analysis of the leukemia cells from a patient with precursor B-ALL demonstrating the expression of CD10, CD34, and HLA-DR by the blast cells.

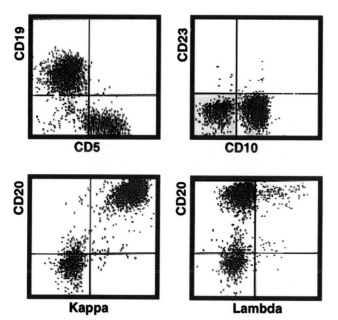

Figure 6–12. Flow cytometric analysis of the leukemia cells from a patient with B-ALL (Burkitt's type) demonstrating the expression of CD10, CD19, and surface kappa light chain by the blast cells.

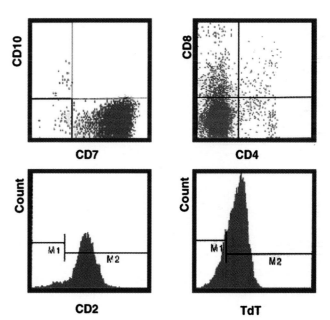

Figure 6–13. Flow cytometric analysis of the leukemia cells from a patient with T-ALL demonstrating expression of CD2, CD7, and TdT by the blast cells. There is no significant expression of CD4 and CD8.

CLINICAL ASPECTS

ALL represents over 75% of all leukemias in children. Clinical symptoms are related to the extent of bone marrow infiltration, severity of cytopenias, and extramedullary involvement. Lymphadenopathy and hepatosplenomegaly are common. Unfavorable prognostic indicators include age younger than 1 and older than 10 years, L3 morphology, massive hepatosplenomegaly, central nervous system (CNS) involvement, hypodiploidy, and t(4; 11) and t(9;22).

DIFFERENTIAL DIAGNOSIS

Differential diagnosis of ALL includes certain subtypes of AML (M0, M1, M5A, M7), Burkitt's and lymphoblastic lymphomas, metastatic small/round cell tumors, and reactive lymphocytosis.

ALL is distinguished from AML by morphology (such as cytoplasmic granules and Auer rods), cytochemical stains, and immunophenotypic features. There is considerable overlap between high-grade lymphomas and ALLs. Some categories of lymphomas, such as lymphoblastic and Burkitt's lymphomas, are considered a clinical spectrum of ALLs. Overall, metastatic round cell tumors are larger than lymphoblasts, and have a tendency to appear in clusters. However, immunophenotypic and ultrastructural studies may be necessary when morphology is equivocal. Viral-induced reactive lymphocytosis is usually a peripheral blood and lymph node process with minimal bone marrow involvement. The reactive lymphocytes are large and pleomorphic, have abundant cytoplasm, often show a coarse nuclear chromatin, and are a mixture of B and T lymphocytes.

Increased numbers of precursor B lymphocytes (hematogones) are seen in the bone marrow samples of young children, post-transplant patients, and patients who are recovering from the bone marrow effects of chemotherapy. Hematogones are positive for CD10, CD19, HLA-DR, and TdT, and therefore may mimic residual leukemia cells in ALL patients undergoing chemotherapy. Hematogones are polyclonal, do not demonstrate cytogenetic abnormalities, and unlike residual ALL cells, usually do not appear in clusters (Figures 6-14 and 6-15).

Selected References

Bennett JM, Catovsky D, Daniel MT, et al: French-American-British (FAB) Cooperative Group proposal for the classification of acute leukemias. Br J Haematol 33:451, 1976.

Bennett JM, Catovsky D, Daniel MT, et al: The morphological classification of acute lymphoblastic leukemia: Concordance among observers and clinical correlations. Br J Haematol 47:553, 1981.

Bezwoda WR, Seymour L, Ariad S, et al: Acute lymphoblastic leukemia in adults. Prognostic factors and 10 year treatment results. Leuk Lymphoma 5:347, 1991.

Borowitz MJ: Immunological markers in childhood acute lymphoblastic leukemia. Hematol Oncol Clin North Am 4:743, 1990.

Davis RE, Langacre TA, Cornbleet PJ: Hematogones in the bone marrow of adults. Am J Clin Pathol 102:207, 1994.

Felix CA, Lange BJ: Leukemia in infants. Oncologist 4:225, 1999.

First MIC Cooperative Study Group: Morphologic, immunologic, and cytogenetic (MIC) working classification of acute lymphoblastic leukemia. Cancer Genet Cytogenet 23:189, 1986.

Fishel RS, Farnen JP, Hanson CA: Acute lymphoblastic leukemia with eosinophilia. Medicine 69:232, 1990.

Groupe Francais de Cytogenetique Hematologique: Cytogenetic abnormalities in adult acute lymphoblastic leukemia: Correlations with hematologic findings and outcome. A collaborative study of the Groupe Francais de Cytogenetique Hematologique. Blood 87:3135, 1996.

Harris NL, Jaffe ES, Diebold J, et al: The World Health Organization classification of hematological malignancies. Report of the Clinical Advisory Committee Meeting. Airlie House, Virginia, November 1997. Mod Pathol 13:193, 2000.

Liang R, Chan TK, Todd D: Childhood acute lymphoblastic leukemia and aplastic anemia. Leuk Lymphoma 13:411, 1994.

Melnick SJ: Acute lymphoblastic leukemia. Clin Lab Medicine 19:169, 1999.

Naeim F: Pathology of Bone Marrow. 2nd ed. Baltimore, Williams & Wilkins, 1998.

Ngan M, Chein K, Lee S: Sudan black B positivity in acute lymphoblastic leukemia. Mod Pathol 5:68, 1992.

Pui C-H, Crist WM: Cytogenetic abnormalities in childhood acute lymphoblastic leukemia correlate with clinical features and treatment outcome. Leuk Lymphoma 7:259, 1992.

Rimsza LM, Viswanatha DS, Winter SS, et al: The presence of CD34+ cell clusters predicts impending relapse in children with acute lymphoblastic leukemia receiving maintenance chemotherapy. Am J Clin Pathol 110:313, 1998.

Traweek ST: Immunophenotypic analysis of acute leukemia. Am J Clin Pathol 99:504, 1993.

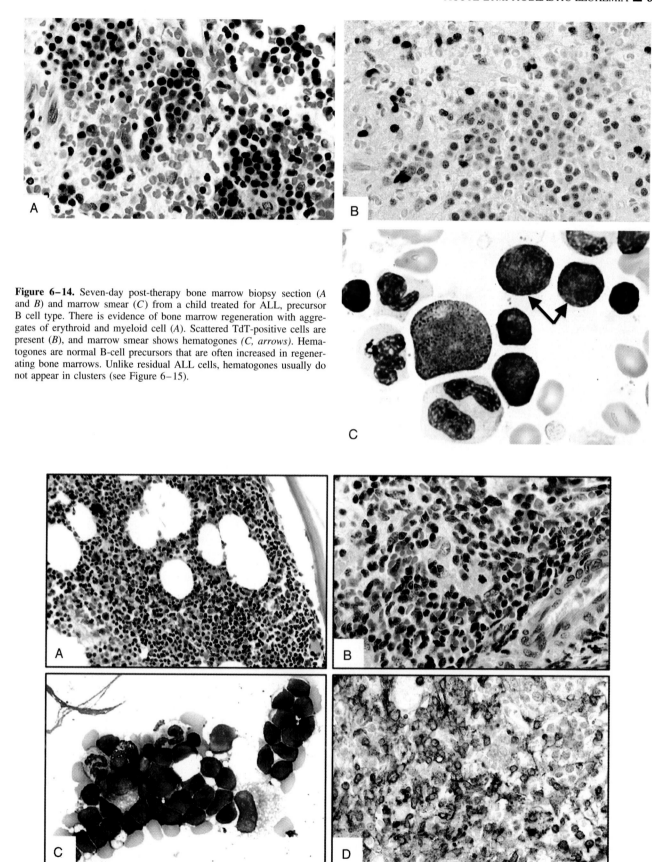

Figure 6–14. Seven-day post-therapy bone marrow biopsy section (*A* and *B*) and marrow smear (*C*) from a child treated for ALL, precursor B cell type. There is evidence of bone marrow regeneration with aggregates of erythroid and myeloid cell (*A*). Scattered TdT-positive cells are present (*B*), and marrow smear shows hematogones *(C, arrows)*. Hematogones are normal B-cell precursors that are often increased in regenerating bone marrows. Unlike residual ALL cells, hematogones usually do not appear in clusters (see Figure 6–15).

Figure 6–15. Seven-day post-therapy bone marrow biopsy section from a child treated for ALL, precursor B cell type. Aggregates of atypical immature lymphoid cells are demonstrated in the bone marrow biopsy section (*A* and *B*, low- and high-power views) and the touch preparation (*C*), representing residual disease. The cells express CD10 (*D*).

CHAPTER 7

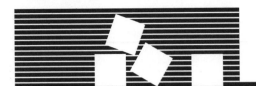

Mixed Lineage Leukemias

The addition of cytochemical, immunophenotypic, cytogenetic, and molecular techniques to the standard morphologic evaluation of the blast cells in acute leukemias has led to a growing incidence of leukemias that share both lymphoid and myeloid features. These leukemias are divided into two major categories: *biphenotypic leukemias* and *bilineal leukemias*. In biphenotypic leukemias, the individual blast cells demonstrate both myeloid and lymphoid features. In bilineal leukemias, two distinct populations of blast cells are present in the same patient. Biphenotypic leukemias are much more frequent than the bilineal ones.

BIPHENOTYPIC LEUKEMIAS

Biphenotypic leukemias are primarily defined by immunophenotypic studies. Differentiation-associated antigens are the main resources for these studies. Since most of these antigens are neither tumor-specific nor lineage-restricted, there is a significant overlap in their expression in myeloid and lymphoid leukemias. Although there are no universally accepted criteria for the inclusion of an acute leukemia in the biphenotypic category, most authors recommend expression of two or more markers of another lineage for the diagnosis of biphenotypic leukemia (Figures 7–1 to 7–3). The most definitive lineage-associated markers are cytoplasmic CD22 and cytoplasmic Igμ for B lymphoblasts, cytoplasmic CD3 for T lymphoblasts, and myeloperoxidase for myeloblasts. In general, based on their clinicopathological features, most biphenotypic leukemias fall into either acute lymphoblastic leukemia (ALL) or acute myelogenous leukemia (AML) subtypes.

Therefore, they could be divided into two major immunophenotypic groups: AMLs expressing lymphoid-associated markers and ALLs expressing myeloid-associated markers.

AMLs Expressing Lymphoid-Associated Markers (Ly+ AMLs)

The leukemia cells, in addition to myeloperoxidase (MPO), Sudan black B (SBB), and/or nonspecific esterase (NSE)- and myeloid-associated antigens, also express lymphoid-associated markers. In some cases, expression of lymphoid markers is associated with specific subtypes of AML or certain cytogenetic abnormalities (Table 7–1). For example, CD19 and TdT are frequently expressed in AMLs with t(11q23) and t(8;21); CD2 is expressed in up to 50% of AML-M3 cases; CD7 is often expressed in AML-M0, -M1, and -M5A; CD56 has been reported in AML-M2 with t(8;21) and in a variant of AML that is morphologically similar to AML-M3 microgranular, but lacks t(15;17).

ALLs Expressing Myeloid-Associated Markers (My+ ALLs)

The blast cells in addition to lymphoid-associated antigens also express myeloid-associated markers, such as CD13, CD14, CD15, CD33, MPO, or SBB. CD15 is frequently expressed in ALLs with t(4;11).

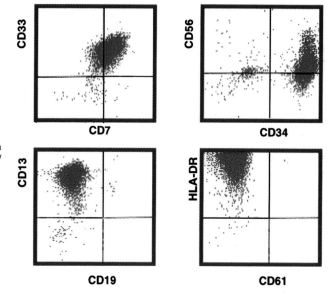

Figure 7–1. Flow cytometric analysis of blast cells in a patient with acute myelogenous leukemia with coexpression of CD7/CD33 and CD34/CD56. Blast cells also express CD13 and HLA-DR.

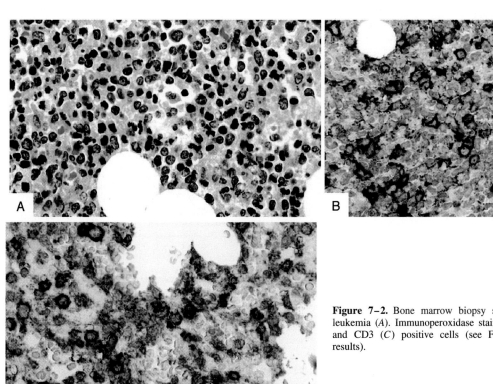

Figure 7–2. Bone marrow biopsy section of a patient with acute leukemia (*A*). Immunoperoxidase stains show a mixture of CD20 (*B*) and CD3 (*C*) positive cells (see Figure 7–3 for flow cytometric results).

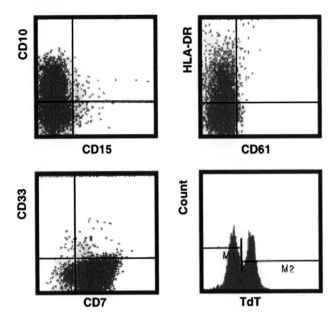

Figure 7–3. Flow cytometric analysis of the blast cells shown in Figure 7–2 demonstrates expression of CD10, HLA-DR, CD7, and TdT, a mixed B- and T-cell phenotype.

Table 7–1
PATHOLOGICAL FEATURES OF Ly$^+$
ACUTE MYELOGENOUS LEUKEMIAS
(AMLs)

Antigen	Frequent Association
TdT	Relatively frequent in AML-M4 and -M5; associated with t(4;11), t(8;21), and t(11;19).
CD2	Associated with AML-M3 microgranular and AML-M4Eo.
CD7	Associated with AML-M0, -M1, and -M5A.
CD19	Associated with t(4;11), t(8;21), and t(11;19).
CD56	Associated with AML-M2 with t(8;21) and expressed in a variant of AML similar to the AML-M3 microgranular but without t(15;17).

BILINEAL LEUKEMIAS

Acute bilineal leukemias, unlike biphenotypic leukemias, are rare and consist of two distinct populations of malignant cells, such as a mixture of myeloblasts and lymphoblasts or a mixture of B lymphoblasts and T lymphoblasts (Figures 7–4 to 7–8).

Selected References

Claxton DF, Reading CL, Nagarajian L, et al: Correlation of CD2 expression with PML gene breakpoints in patients with acute promyelocytic leukemia. Blood 80:582, 1992.

Cuneo A, Michaux J-L, Ferrant A, et al: Correlation of cytogenetic patterns and clinicobiological features in adult acute myeloid leukemia expressing lymphoid markers. Blood 79:720, 1992.

Drexler HG, Sperling C, Leudwig W-D: Terminal deoxynucleotidyl transferase (TdT) expression in acute myeloid leukemia. Leukemia 7:1142, 1993.

Hurwitz CA, Raimondi SC, Head D, et al: Distinctive immunophenotypic features of t(8;21)(q22;q22) acute myeloblastic leukemia in children. Blood 80:3182, 1992.

Kuerbitz SJ, Civin CI, Krischer JP, et al: Expression of myeloid-associated and lymphoid-associated cell-surface antigens in acute myeloid leukemia of childhood. A Pediatric Oncology group study. J Clin Oncol 10:1419, 1992.

Matutes E, Morilla R, Farahat N, et al: Definition of acute biphenotypic leukemia. Haematologica 82:64, 1997.

Neame PB, Soamboonsrup P, Browman GP, et al: Simultaneous or sequential expression of lymphoid and myeloid phenotypes in acute leukemia. Blood 65:142, 1985.

Pui C-H, Raimondi SC, Head DR, et al: Characterization of childhood acute leukemia with multiple myeloid and lymphoid markers at diagnosis and at relapse. Blood 78:1327, 1991.

Stass SA, Mirro J: Lineage heterogeneity in acute leukaemia: acute mixed-lineage switch. Clin Haematol 15:811, 1986.

Suzuki R, Yamamoto K, Seto M, et al: CD7+ and CD56+ myeloid/natural killer cell precursor acute leukemia: A distinct hematolymphoid disease entity. Blood 90:2417, 1997.

Traweek ST: Immunophenotypic analysis of acute leukemia. Am J Clin Pathol 99:504, 1993.

Ueda T, Kita K, Kagawa D, et al: Acute leukemia with two cell populations of lymphoblasts and monoblasts. Leuk Res 8:63, 1984.

Unkun M, Sather HN, Gaynon PS, et al: Clinical features and treatment outcome of children with myeloid antigen positive acute lymphoblastic lymphoma: A report from the Children's Cancer Group. Blood 90:28, 1997.

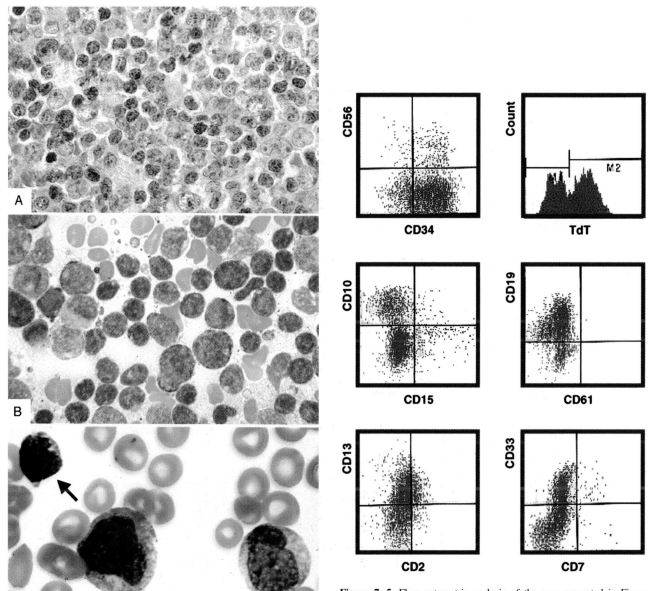

Figure 7–5. Flow cytometric analysis of the case presented in Figure 7–4. Leukemia cells are mostly CD34-positive, but some express CD10, CD19, and TdT, and some are CD13- and CD33-positive.

Figure 7–4. Bone marrow biopsy section (*A*) and marrow smear (*B*) demonstrating two blast populations: The small blasts are lymphoid, and the large blasts are myeloid in origin. Blood smear (*C*) shows a lymphoblast *(arrow)* and a type II myeloblast (center). Flow cytometric analysis (see Figure 7–5) depicted two separate blast populations.

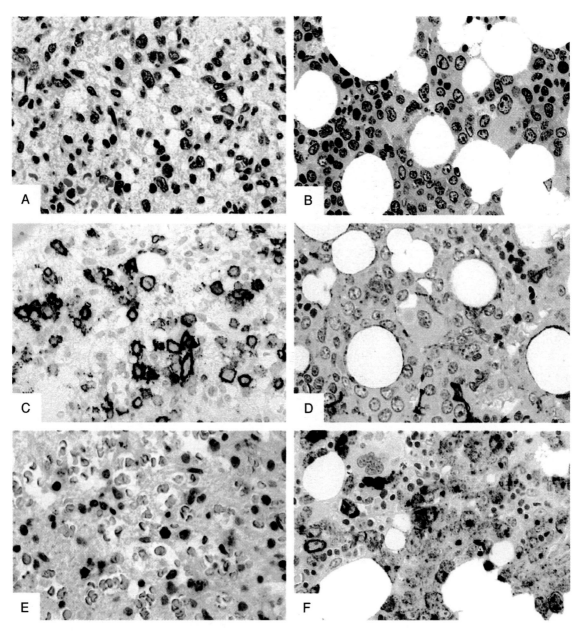

Figure 7–6. Post-therapy bone marrow biopsy sections from a patient with a history of bilineage acute leukemia (AML/ALL). Figures in the left column, *A, C,* and *E,* represent residual ALL after the first post-therapy sample. Small clusters of CD10-positive cells are present (*C*), whereas only occasional cells are positive for myeloperoxidase (*E*). Figures in the right column, *B, D,* and *F,* represent residual AML after the second round of chemotherapy. This time, rare CD10-positive cells are present (*D*), whereas numerous cells are positive for myeloperoxidase (*F*).

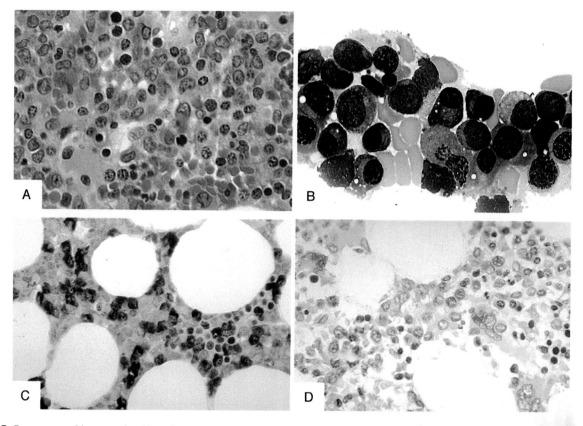

Figure 7–7. Bone marrow biopsy section (*A*) and marrow smear (*B*) from a patient with a combination of AML and plasma cell dyscrasia. Plasma cells express Ig lambda light chain (*C*) and are negative for Ig kappa light chain (*D*).

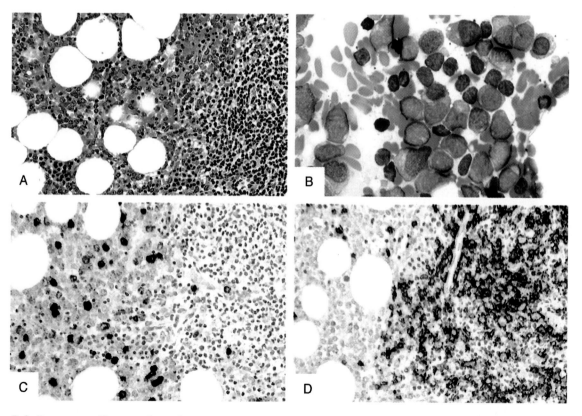

Figure 7–8. Bone marrow biopsy section and marrow smear demonstrating a combination of AML and non-Hodgkin's lymphoma. An interstitial infiltrate of blast cells and an atypical lymphoid aggregate are seen in the biopsy section (*A*). Marrow smear demonstrates a mixture of myeloblasts and atypical lymphocytes (*B*). Immunohistochemical stains on the biopsy section reveal myeloperoxidase-positive blast cells (*C*) and a lymphoid aggregate strongly expressing CD20 (*D*). The patient had a diagnosis of follicular lymphoma 4 years ago and was treated with chemotherapy. Recently, he developed generalized lymphadenopathy and pancytopenia.

CHAPTER 8

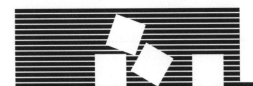

Chronic Lymphoid
Leukemias

Chronic lymphoid leukemias are the results of mono-clonal proliferation of mature-appearing lymphocytes representing several well-defined clinicopathologic entities, such as chronic lymphocytic leukemia (CLL), prolymphocytic leukemia (PLL), hairy cell leukemia (HCL), Sézary syndrome, and adult T-cell leukemia/lymphoma (ATLL) (Table 8–1). The overwhelming majority of chronic lymphoid leukemias are of the B-cell type. The T-cell variant is mostly of CD4⁺ phenotype.

Table 8–1
MAJOR SUBCLASSES OF CHRONIC (MATURE) LYMPHOID LEUKEMIAS

Type	Morphology	Main Cell Markers
CLL	Small mature lymphocytes with scanty cytoplasm	>99% B cell: CD5, CD19, CD20, CD23, CD24, and weak SmIg
PLL	Prolymphocytes, intermediate to large cells, variable amount of cytoplasm, and prominent nucleolus	>80% B cell: CD19, CD20, CD22, and strong SmIg
HCL	Intermediate to large cells, abundant cytoplasm with cytoplasmic projections	>99% B cell: TRAP, CD19, CD20, CD22, CD25, CD103, CD11c, and strong SmIg
LGLL	Intermediate to large cells, abundant cytoplasm with cytoplasmic azurophilic granules	T cell or NK cell type: CD16, CD56, CD57, TIA-1 T-cell type: CD3⁺/CD8⁺ NK-cell type: CD3⁻/CD8⁺
ATLL	Small to large cells, irregular nuclei with rough nuclear convolutions	Helper T cell: CD2, CD3, CD4, CD5, CD25, HTLV-1
Sézary	Small to large cells, irregular nuclei with fine nuclear convolutions	Helper T cell: CD2, CD3, CD4, CD5

CLL = chronic lymphoid leukemia; SmIg = surface membrane Ig; PLL = prolymphocytic leukemia; HCL = hairy cell leukemia; LGLL = large granular lymphocytic leukemia; ATLL = adult T-cell leukemia/lymphoma; NK = natural killer; TRAP = tartrate-resistant acid phosphatase; HTLV = human T-cell lymphotrophic virus.

CHRONIC LYMPHOCYTIC LEUKEMIA

The National Cancer Institute–Sponsored Workshop Group has proposed certain criteria for the diagnosis of CLL. These criteria include: (1) a peripheral lymphocyte count of more than 5000/μL; (2) bone marrow lymphocytosis of 30% or greater (Figures 8–1 to 8–5); and the coexpression of B cell–associated markers (CD19, CD20, CD23) and CD5 by the lymphocytes (Figure 8–6). Establishment of a diagnosis in rare cases may require evidence of monoclonality by immunophenotypic and or molecular studies. Over 99% of the CLLs are of B-cell type.

The CLL cells are typically small with scanty dark blue nongranular cytoplasm, round nucleus, dense chromatin, and inconspicuous or invisible nucleoli (see Figures 8–1 to 8–5). However, rare cases of CLL may show larger cells with more cytoplasm or cells with irregular or indented nuclei. Prolymphocytes are a frequent component of CLL but usually do not exceed 10% of the tumor cells. The bone marrow involvement is usually interstitial or diffuse, but patchy or nodular patterns are occasionally seen. Approximately 5% of the CLL cases may lack expression of CD5 and/or CD23. CLL cells express a relatively low concentration of surface immunoglobulin (Ig), but the Ig expression when detected is monoclonal.

Most frequent cytogenetic abnormalities in CLL are trisomy 12, and structural abnormalities in chromosomes 13(q14) and 14(q32).

CLL and small lymphocytic lymphoma (see Chapter 9) share wide clinicopathologic features and appear to represent different spectrums of the same disorder, one with primary involvement of the bone marrow and blood, and the other with primary involvement of the lymph nodes.

Chronic Lymphocytic Leukemia Variants

CLL, mixed cell type, is a term proposed by the French-American-British (FAB) Cooperative Group for the cases that are composed of a mixture of small and large lymphoid cells (Figures 8–7 to 8–9). Some of the cases consist of mature lymphocytes and prolymphocytes, with prolymphocytes accounting for between 10% and 55% of the tumor cells. These cases are referred to as *CLL/PLL* (see Figures 8–7 and 8–8). The term *atypical CLL* is used to indicate unusual morphologic (variation in size, nuclear irregularity) features (see Figure 8–9) or immunophenotypic patterns (lack of CD5 and/or CD23). Occasional cases of CLL consist of larger cells with abundant cytoplasm, resembling hairy cell leukemia. However, these cells, unlike hairy cells, are negative for tartrate-resistant acid phosphatase (TRAP) and do not express CD103.

T-CLL, a rare entity (<1% of CLLs), is characterized by marked lymphocytosis and frequent involvement of extramedullary tissues. T-CLL is usually of helper/inducer (CD4+) phenotype. In the recently proposed World Health Organization (WHO) classification, T-CLL is considered a variant of T-cell prolymphocytic leukemia.

Chronic Lymphocytic Leukemia Transformation

Ten to thirty percent of the patients with CLL eventually develop a more aggressive lymphoid malignancy. This development, in most instances, is the result of transformation of the CLL cells to blast or other lymphoid cells, but it may also represent a second malignant clone. Development of prolymphocytic leukemia and non-Hodgkin's large cell lymphoma (Richter's syndrome) has been reported in 30% and 10% of the CLL patients, respectively (Figures 8–10 and 8–11). Hodgkin's disease, multiple myeloma and acute lymphoblastic leukemia (ALL) are other examples of lymphoid malignancies that occasionally evolve in patients with CLL (Figure 8–12).

Clinical Aspects

CLL accounts for approximately 30% of adult leukemias in Western countries. The median age of incidence is 55 with a male:female ratio of 2 to 3:1. Extensive extramedullary involvement, low hemoglobin levels (<10g/dL), and thrombocytopenia (platelet count <100,000/μL) are associated with poor prognosis.

Differential Diagnosis

Differential diagnosis of CLL includes prolymphocytic leukemia, hairy cell leukemia, mantle cell lymphoma, small cleaved follicular lymphoma, and persistent polyclonal B lymphocytosis. CLL consists of lymphocytes with scanty cytoplasm and regular nuclei; prolymphocytes are less than 10% of the cells in the typical CLL and less than 55% in the CLL/PLL variant. CLL cells are TRAP- and CD103-negative, express CD5 and B cell–associated antigens including CD23, but are CD10-negative (see Figure 8–6).

Persistent polyclonal B lymphocytosis is a rare condition reported in middle-aged women who are heavy smokers. Its morphologic hallmark is the presence of binucleated lymphocytes and lack of bone marrow lymphocytosis (see Chapter 13).

Text continued on page 105

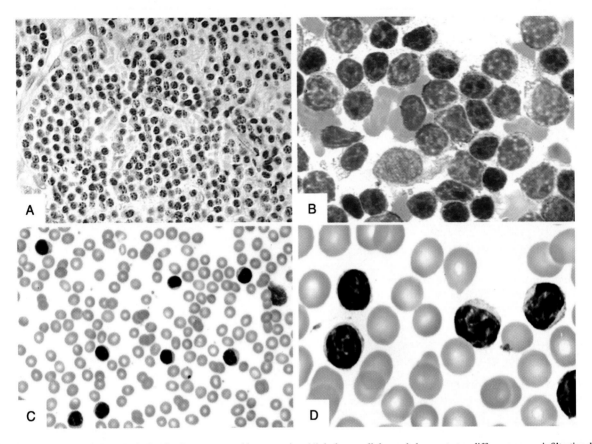

Figure 8–1. Chronic lymphocytic leukemia. Bone marrow biopsy section (*A*) is hypercellular and demonstrates diffuse marrow infiltration by small lymphocytes. Blue-stained granules are iron particles. Smears from bone marrow (*B*) and blood (*C* and *D*) show increased numbers of lymphocytes. Most of the lymphocytes have scanty cytoplasm, round or slightly irregular nuclei, condensed nuclear chromatin, and inconspicuous nucleoli.

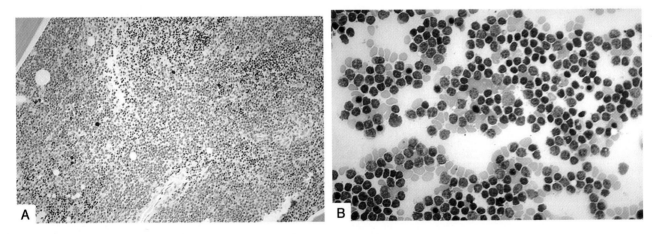

Figure 8–2. Chronic lymphocytic leukemia. Bone marrow biopsy section (*A*) is hypercellular and demonstrates diffuse marrow infiltration by small lymphocytes. Bone marrow smear (*B*) shows sheets of small lymphocytes. Most of the lymphocytes have scanty cytoplasm, round or slightly irregular nuclei, condensed nuclear chromatin, and inconspicuous nucleoli. (*B*, from Naeim F: Pathology of Bone Marrow, 2nd ed. Baltimore, WIlliams & Wilkins, 1998, with permission.)

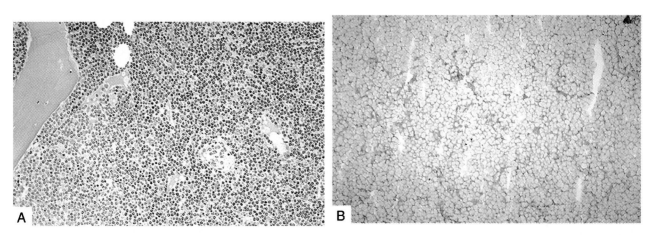

Figure 8–3. Chronic lymphocytic leukemia. Bone marrow biopsy sections are hypercellular and show a diffuse lymphocytic infiltration (*A*) with the expression of CD20 (*B*, immunoperoxidase stain).

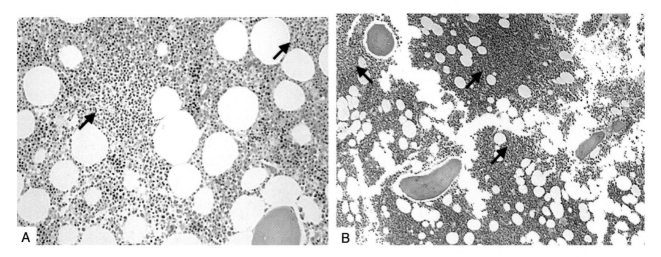

Figure 8–4. Chronic lymphocytic leukemia. Bone marrow biopsy sections demonstrate several lymphoid aggregates of small mature lymphocytes. The aggregates are in various shapes and sizes (*A* and *B, arrows*).

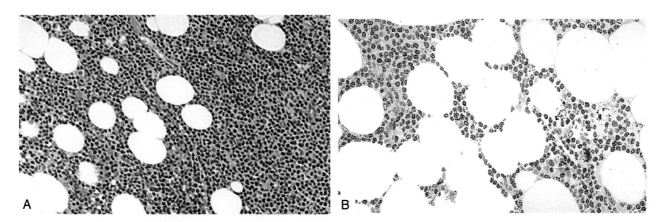

Figure 8–5. Chronic lymphocytic leukemia. Bone marrow biopsy sections demonstrate various patterns of lymphoid infiltration: a mixed diffuse and interstitial pattern (*A*) and an interstitial pattern (*B*).

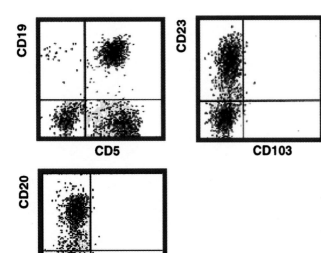

Figure 8–6. Flow cytometric analysis of lymphocytes in a patient with chronic lymphocytic leukemia. The leukemia cells coexpress CD5 and CD19, are positive for CD20 and CD23, and do not express CD10 and CD103.

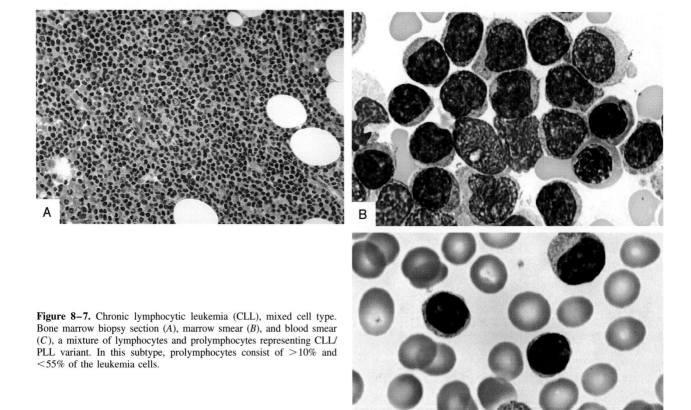

Figure 8–7. Chronic lymphocytic leukemia (CLL), mixed cell type. Bone marrow biopsy section (*A*), marrow smear (*B*), and blood smear (*C*), a mixture of lymphocytes and prolymphocytes representing CLL/PLL variant. In this subtype, prolymphocytes consist of >10% and <55% of the leukemia cells.

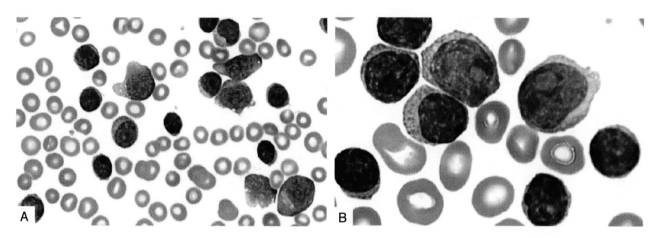

Figure 8–8. Chronic lymphocytic leukemia, mixed cell type. *A* and *B*, Blood smears demonstrate a mixture of lymphocytes and prolymphocytes representing CLL/PLL variant.

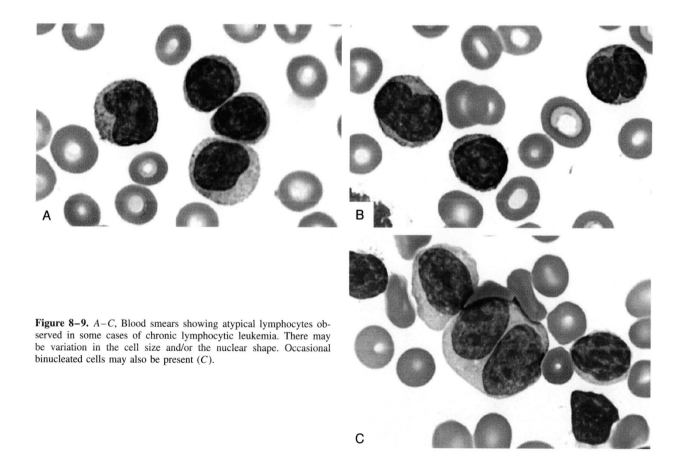

Figure 8–9. *A–C*, Blood smears showing atypical lymphocytes observed in some cases of chronic lymphocytic leukemia. There may be variation in the cell size and/or the nuclear shape. Occasional binucleated cells may also be present (*C*).

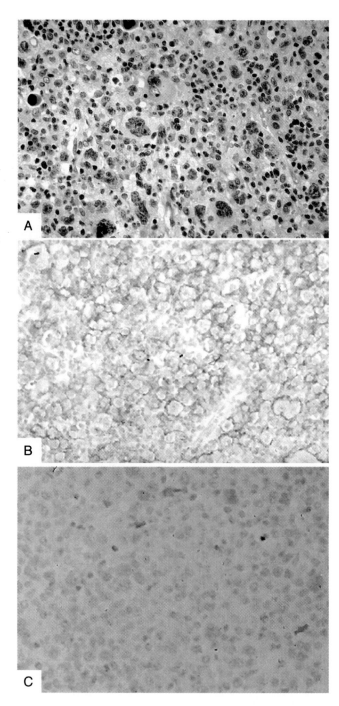

Figure 8–10. Chronic lymphocytic leukemia in blast transformation (Richter's syndrome). Lymph node sections (*A* and *B*) demonstrating a mixed population of small and large cells. The large cells have a variable amount of cytoplasm with large nuclei and prominent nucleoli (*B, arrow*). Immunoperoxidase stain demonstrates several CD30-positive large cells (*C, arrow*).

Figure 8–11. Transformation of CLL to anaplastic large cell lymphoma. Lymph node section (*A*) from a patient with a longstanding history of CLL demonstrates numerous large cells, including large bizarre forms with nuclear lobulation or multiple nuclei. The overall features resemble Hodgkin's lymphoma. However, the large cells express CD20 (*B*) and are negative for CD30 (*C*). The same cells also expressed Ig kappa light chain (results not shown). Findings are consistent with an anaplastic large B-cell lymphoma. (From Naeim F: Pathology of Bone Marrow, 2nd ed. Baltimore, Williams & Wilkins, 1998, with permission.)

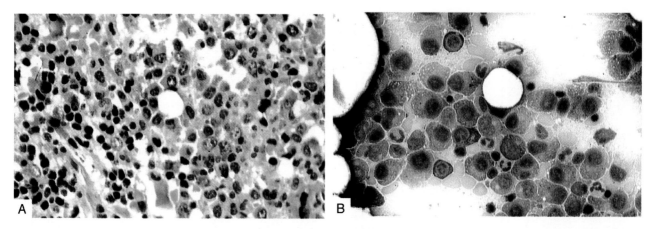

Figure 8–12. Development of plasma cell myeloma in a patient with a history of CLL. Bone marrow biopsy section (*A*) and marrow smear (*B*) show sheets of atypical plasma cells. Residual CLL is evident in the left lower part of the biopsy section (*A*).

PROLYMPHOCYTIC LEUKEMIA

Prolymphocytic leukemia (PLL) is characterized by marked peripheral blood lymphocytosis (usually >100,000/μL), with the presence of 55% or more prolymphocytes. Prolymphocytes are larger than CLL cells, and display a variable amount of cytoplasm, round or irregular nuclei, condensed chromatin, and one prominent nucleolus (Figures 8–13 to 8–15). The bone marrow involvement, similar to CLL, may be focal, interstitial, diffuse, or a combination of these.

PLL cells in approximately 80% of the cases are of B-cell origin and express CD19, CD20, and CD22, and often a strong monoclonal membrane Ig. They are negative for CD5, CD10, and CD23. Prolymphocytes in the T-cell variant are of helper/inducer (CD4$^+$) phenotype (Figure 8–16).

The most frequent cytogenetic abnormalities in PLL involve chromosomes 6 and 14, including 6q−, 14q+, t(6;12), and t(11;14).

Clinical Aspects

PLL is less frequent than CLL and on the average patients are older (about 50% of the patients are over 70 years old). Marked splenomegaly and absent or minimal lymphadenopathy are the major clinical findings.

Differential Diagnosis

Differential diagnosis of PLL includes HCL and CLL variants, blastic variant of mantle cell lymphoma, acute monocytic leukemia, and large cell lymphoma. PLL cells are negative for CD5, CD10, CD23, BCL-1, TRAP, and monocytic markers (such as CD14, CD64, and CD68), and strongly express CD22, FMC7, and membrane Ig. Marked lymphocytosis and absent or minimal lymphadenopathy distinguishes PLL from large cell lymphomas.

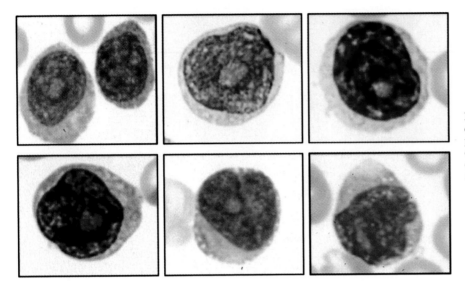

Figure 8–13. Prolymphocytes. Prolympho-cytes are larger than lymphocytes and dis-play a variable amount of cytoplasm, round or irregular nuclei, condensed chromatin, and one prominent nucleolus. Some may contain a few azurophilic granules.

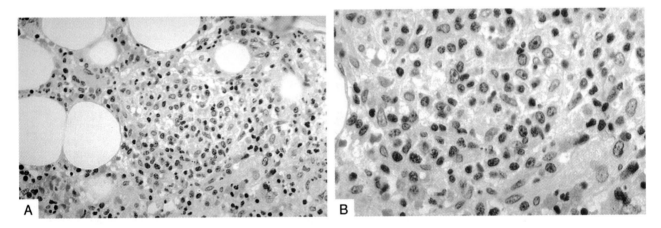

Figure 8–14. Prolymphocytic leukemia. Bone marrow biopsy section demonstrates an aggregate of prolymphocytes (low-power [A] and high-power [B] views). The prolymphocytes show a variable amount of cytoplasm, which creates an uneven nuclear spacing. The nuclei are round or irregular, and many cells show a single prominent nucleolus.

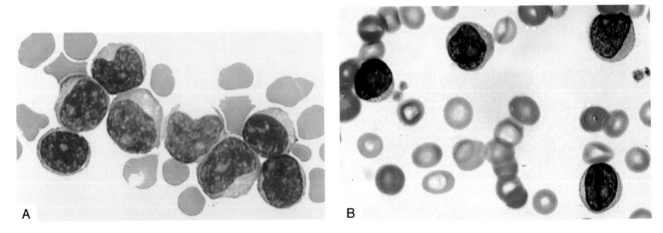

Figure 8–15. Prolymphocytic leukemia. Bone marrow (A) and blood (B) smears demonstrate several promyelocytes. (A, from Naeim F: Pathology of Bone Marrow, 2nd ed. Baltimore, Williams & Wilkins, 1998, with permission.)

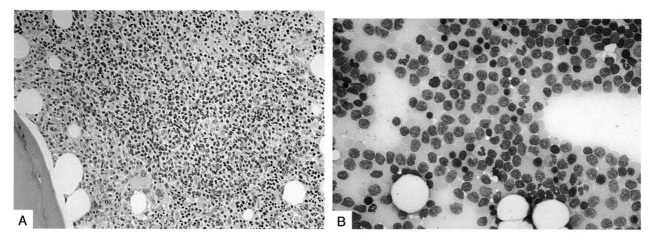

Figure 8–16. Prolymphocytic leukemia. Bone marrow biopsy section (*A*) and marrow smear (*B*) demonstrate sheets of promyelocytes. The majority of the prolymphocytes show slight nuclear irregularity. Immunophenotypic studies showed expression of CD2, CD3, and CD4, consistent with a T-cell variant of prolymphocytic leukemia (results not shown).

HAIRY CELL LEUKEMIA

Hairy cell leukemia is a chronic lymphoid leukemia characterized by the proliferation of lymphocytes with cytoplasmic "hairy" projections involving blood, bone marrow, spleen, and occasionally other tissues (see Figures 8–17 to 8–20). Hairy cells are larger than lymphocytes and show abundant pale blue cytoplasm with elongated (hairy) cytoplasmic projections (see Figures 8–19 and 8–20). The nuclei are usually round or oval, but may display folding, indentation, or lobulation (see Figures 8–19 and 8–20). Nuclear chromatin is finer than the CLL cells and nucleoli are usually inconspicuous. Hairy cells are positive for TRAP and express B cell–associated markers (CD19, CD20, CD22, FMC7), as well as CD25, CD103, HLA-DR, and monoclonal membrane Ig (Figures 8–21 and 8–22). They are usually negative for CD5, CD10, and CD23, and display abundant adhesion molecules (CD11c and CD18).

In blood, hairy cells range widely from as low as 5% to over 50% of the white blood cell count (WBC). Pancytopenia is a common feature with marked monocytopenia. Bone marrow involvement is usually interstitial or diffuse. The infiltrating hairy cells show abundant clear cytoplasm, creating wide nuclear spacing. Bone marrow is often hypercellular, but in occasional cases is markedly hypocellular, resembling aplastic anemia (Figures 8–23 to 8–25). Bone marrow reticulin fibrosis is a frequent feature, causing a high rate (>50%) of unsuccessful marrow aspiration (dry tap) in these patients (see Figure 8–23). Sections of spleen show a diffuse red pulp involvement with hairy cells (see Figure 8–18*A*).

Common cytogenetic abnormalities include trisomy of chromosomes 3, 4, 5, 12, and 18, as well as 6q− and 11q−.

Hairy Cell Leukemia Subtypes

HCL variant (HCL-V) displays hairy cells with morphologic features of prolymphocytes (such as prominent nucleolus) (Figures 8–26 and 8–27). The HCL-V is rare and is usually associated with markedly elevated WBC (>50,000/μL) and lack of CD25 expression by the tumor cells. Also, occasional cases of HCL may show hairy cells with multilobated nuclei. A blastic variant of HCL has been reported with TRAP-positive blast-like hairy cells.

Clinical Aspects

The average age of the patients with HCL is around 50 years with a male:female ratio of 3 to 5:1. Lymphadenopathy is infrequent, but splenomegaly and hepatomegaly are common.

Differential Diagnosis

The differential diagnosis of HCL includes marginal zone B-cell lymphoma (splenic lymphoma with villous lymphocytes, monocytoid B-cell lymphoma), CLL variants, and mastocytosis. Marginal zone B-cell lymphoma is negative for TRAP and CD103. Bone marrow mastocytosis may show nuclear spacing and fibrosis resembling HCL. However, mast cells contain cytoplasmic granules (positive by toluidine blue, Giemsa, and chloroacetate stains), do not express B-cell markers, and are negative for TRAP and CD103.

Text continued on page 113

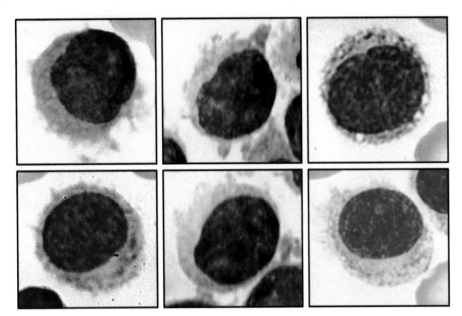

Figure 8–17. Hairy cells. Hairy cells are larger than lymphocytes and show abundant pale blue cytoplasm and cytoplasmic projections. The nuclei are usually round or oval but may display folding or indentation. Nuclear chromatin is slightly finer than in the CLL cells, and nucleoli are usually inconspicuous.

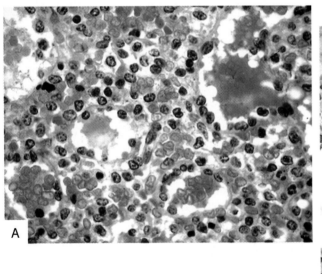

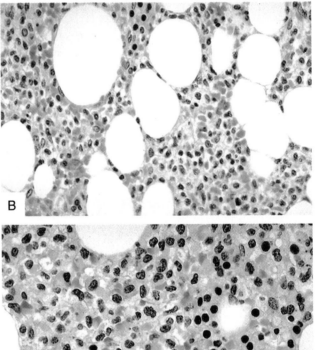

Figure 8–18. Hairy cell leukemia. Spleen and bone marrow are the most frequent organs involved with hairy cell leukemia. Infiltration of the spleen is diffuse and involves the splenic red pulp (A). Bone marrow biopsy sections often show an interstitial involvement (low-power [B] and high-power [C] views).

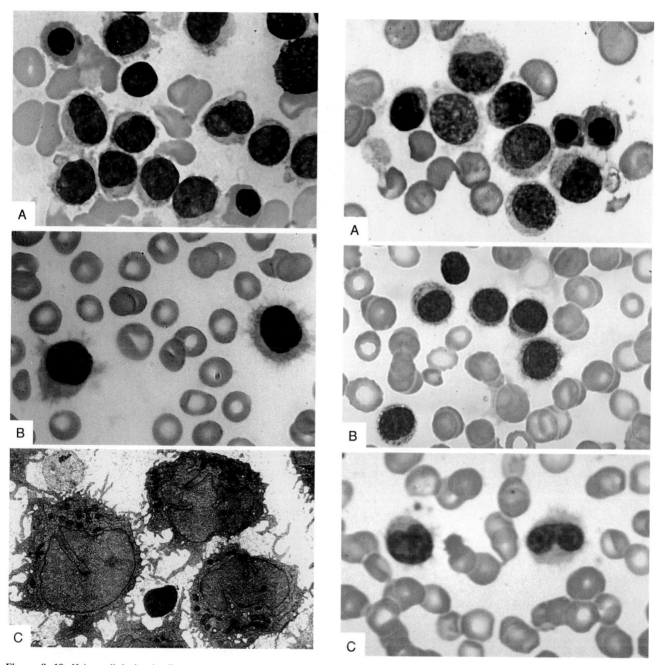

Figure 8–19. Hairy cell leukemia. Bone marrow (*A*) and blood (*B*) smears show hairy cells with cytoplasmic projections and variation in nuclear shape. Electron micrograph of hairy cells demonstrates elongated cytoplasmic projections (*C*).

Figure 8–20. Hairy cell leukemia. Bone marrow (*A*) and blood (*B* and *C*) smears demonstrate hairy cells with cytoplasmic projections and variation in nuclear shape.

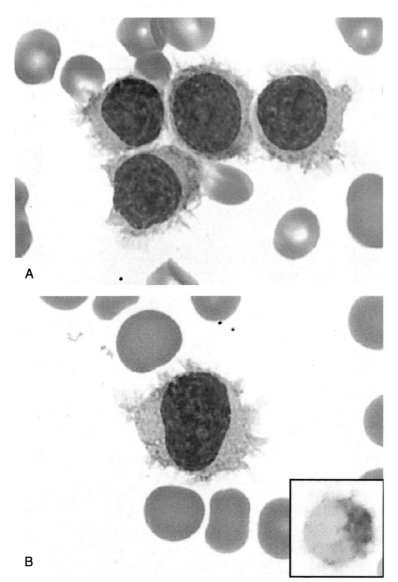

A

B

Figure 8–21. Hairy cell leukemia. Blood smears (*A* and *B*) demonstrate hairy cells with cytoplasmic projections. The inset shows a hairy cell staining for tartrate-resistant acid phosphatase (TRAP).

Figure 8–22. Hairy cell leukemia. Flow cytometry of hairy cells demonstrates expression of CD11c, CD22, FMC7, CD25, and CD103.

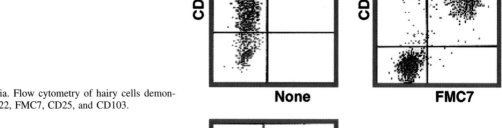

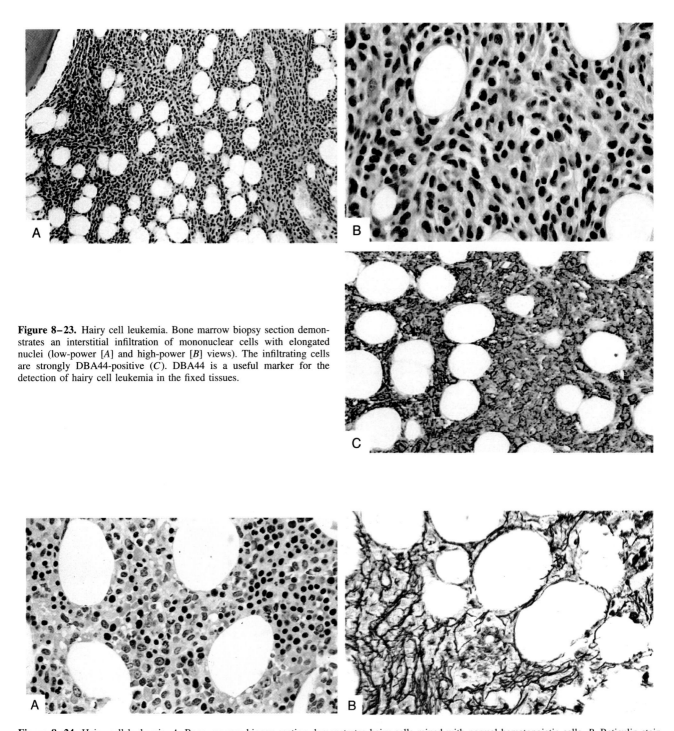

Figure 8–23. Hairy cell leukemia. Bone marrow biopsy section demonstrates an interstitial infiltration of mononuclear cells with elongated nuclei (low-power [A] and high-power [B] views). The infiltrating cells are strongly DBA44-positive (C). DBA44 is a useful marker for the detection of hairy cell leukemia in the fixed tissues.

Figure 8–24. Hairy cell leukemia. A, Bone marrow biopsy section demonstrates hairy cells mixed with normal hematopoietic cells. B, Reticulin stain shows marked increase in reticulin fibers.

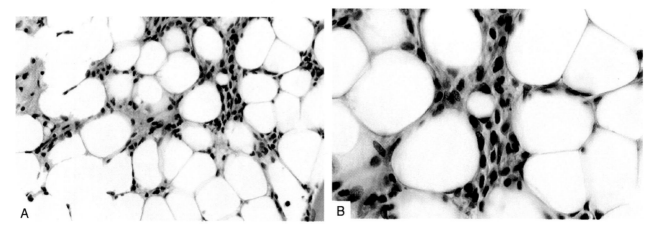

Figure 8–25. Hairy cell leukemia. The hypocellular variant of hairy cell leukemia may resemble aplastic anemia in bone marrow biopsy sections. Interstitial or focal hairy cell infiltration is sometimes overlooked (*A* and *B*).

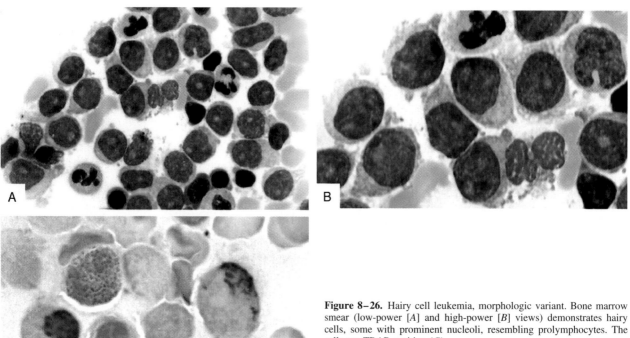

Figure 8–26. Hairy cell leukemia, morphologic variant. Bone marrow smear (low-power [*A*] and high-power [*B*] views) demonstrates hairy cells, some with prominent nucleoli, resembling prolymphocytes. The cells are TRAP-positive (*C*).

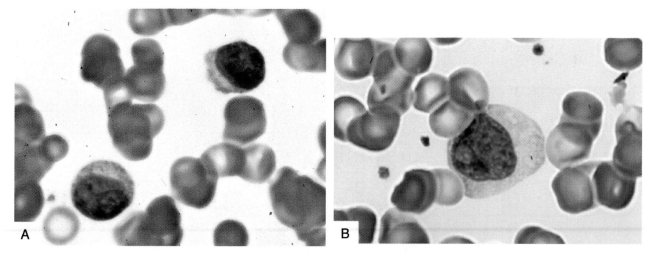

Figure 8–27. Hairy cell leukemia, morphologic variants, blood smears. Hairy cells may occasionally contain cytoplasmic granules (*A*) or may resemble prolymphocytes (*B*). These variants are TRAP-positive and often express CD103.

LARGE GRANULAR LYMPHOCYTIC LEUKEMIA

Large granular lymphocytic leukemia (LGLL) represents monoclonal proliferation of the large granular lymphocytes. These cells are larger than the typical mature lymphocytes and have moderate to abundant cytoplasm with numerous azurophilic granules (Figure 8–28). These granules contain cytolytic enzymes, such as perforin and granzyme. The nucleus is round or oval with condensed chromatin and inconspicuous nucleoli. There are no universally accepted criteria for the diagnosis of LGLL, but in general, persistent idiopathic large granular lymphocytosis (for at least 6 months after the initial presentation) evidenced by absolute count ($>1 \times 1^6/\mu$L) and/or elevated proportion ($>25\%$) by differential count are primary characteristics of LGLL. Enumeration of the large granular lymphocytes is based on morphologic and/or immunophenotypic features (expression of CD16, CD56, CD57, and TIA-1) (Figures 8–29 to 8–31).

Bone marrow involvement is frequent and the pattern of involvement may vary from focal to interstitial or diffuse (see Figures 8–29 and 8–30). Marrow smears show increased numbers of large granular lymphocytes.

Classification

There are two types of LGLL: T-cell type (T-LGLL) and natural killer type (NK-LGLL) (see Figure 8–31). The T-cell type is CD3$^+$, often represents the suppressor/cytotoxic phenotype (CD8$^+$), and demonstrates T-cell receptor (TCR) gene rearrangement. The NK type is CD3-negative and does not reveal TCR gene rearrangement. Both types express one or more of the NK-associated antigens, such as CD16, CD56, and/or CD57, and react positively with antibodies raised against granzyme/perforin granules, such as TIA-1.

Clinical Aspects

The median age at onset is about 55 years for T-LGLL and 40 years for NK-LGLL. There is strong association between T-LGLL and the triad of rheumatoid arthritis, neutropenia, and splenomegaly. Overall, NK-LGLL patients are less neutropenic, but show more severe anemia and thrombocytopenia than patients with T-LGLL. Predictors of aggressive clinical course include age under 40, organomegaly, and CD56$^+$ phenotype.

Differential Diagnosis

Differential diagnosis of LGLL includes chronic reactive large granular lymphocytosis. Relative or absolute large granular lymphocytosis has been observed in viral infections and in association with other malignancies, such as multiple myeloma and CLL.

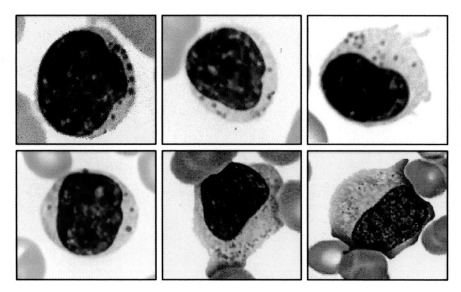

Figure 8–28. Large granular lymphocytes. These cells are larger than the typical mature lymphocytes and have moderate to abundant cytoplasm with numerous azurophilic granules. The granules contain cytolytic enzymes, such as perforin and granzyme. The nucleus is round or oval with condensed chromatin and inconspicuous nuclei. Some of the reactive lymphocytes are of the granular type (bottom, middle and right).

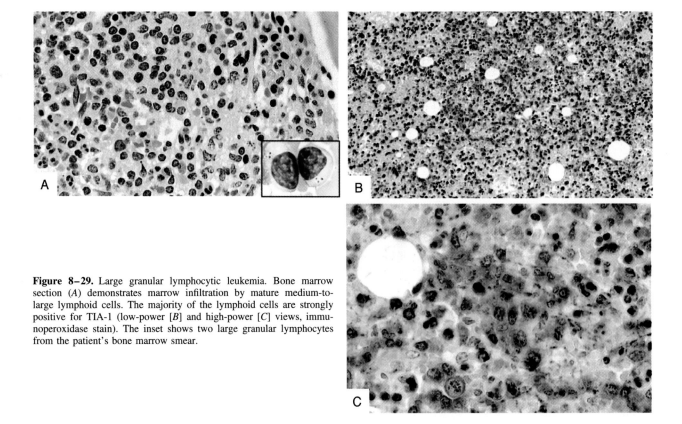

Figure 8–29. Large granular lymphocytic leukemia. Bone marrow section (*A*) demonstrates marrow infiltration by mature medium-to-large lymphoid cells. The majority of the lymphoid cells are strongly positive for TIA-1 (low-power [*B*] and high-power [*C*] views, immunoperoxidase stain). The inset shows two large granular lymphocytes from the patient's bone marrow smear.

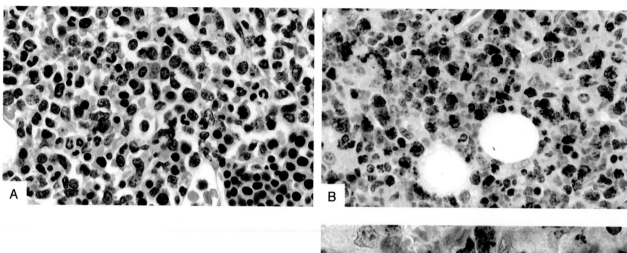

Figure 8–30. Large granular lymphocytic leukemia. Bone marrow section (*A*) demonstrates marrow infiltration by mature medium-to-large lymphoid cells. The majority of the lymphoid cells are strongly positive for TIA-1 (low-power [*B*] and high-power [*C*] views, immunoperoxidase stain).

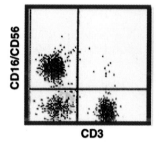 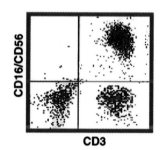

Figure 8–31. Large granular lymphocytic leukemia is divided into two major categories: NK-cell and T-cell types. The NK-cell type is CD16/CD56-positive and CD3-negative (left), and the T-cell type is CD16/CD56- and CD3-positive (right).

ADULT T-CELL LEUKEMIA/LYMPHOMA

Adult T-cell leukemia/lymphoma (ATLL) is a monoclonal lymphoproliferative disorder associated with type 1 human T-cell lymphotrophic virus (HTLV-1).

The ATLL cells are pleomorphic, vary in size, display a variable amount of basophilic cytoplasm, and show marked nuclear convolution ("flower" or "clover leaf" cells) (Figure 8–32). The nuclear chromatin is condensed and the nucleoli are inconspicuous. The ATLL cells are of helper/inducer (CD4$^+$) T cells and also express CD2, CD3, CD5, and CD25. They are negative for CD7 and TdT.

Bone marrow involvement may range from small and focal to massive and diffuse infiltration by atypical lymphocytes with convoluted nuclei.

The most frequent cytogenetic abnormalities in ATLL are 14q−, trisomy 3, 7, or 21, and loss of chromosome X.

Clinical Aspects

ATLL is observed as an endemic disease in the adult population of southwestern Japan. It also affects non-Japanese people, particularly African Americans in the southwestern United States and the Caribbean. The reported median age in the United States is about 35. ATLL is extremely rare in children.

Symptomatic patients often show hepatosplenomegaly, lymphadenopathy, and skin involvement. Poor prognostic factors include age older than 40 years, hypercalcemia, elevated lactate dehydrogenase (LDH), and massive tissue/organ involvement.

Differential Diagnosis

Sézary syndrome and other lymphoproliferative disorders with convoluted nuclei are included in the differential diagnosis of ATLL (see Table 8–1). The nuclear convolution is much more pronounced in ATLL cells than other lymphoid malignancies. Unlike Sézary cells, ATLL cells are HTLV-1–positive, and express CD25.

Sézary Syndrome

Sézary syndrome (leukemic phase of cutaneous T-cell lymphoma, mycosis fungoides) is a chronic T-cell lymphoproliferative disorder characterized by atypical lymphocytes with fine (cerebriform) nuclear convolution (Figures 8–33 and 8–34). The tumor cells (Sézary cells) vary in size, and show scanty blue cytoplasm with no azurophilic granules. The nuclear chromatin is condensed and the nucleoli are inconspicuous. The Sézary cells are of helper/inducer (CD4$^+$) phenotype, are positive for CD2, CD3, and CD5, but typically lack CD7, CD25, TdT, and HLA-DR expression. Sézary cells frequently display DNA hyperdiploidy and sometimes show coexpression of CD4 and CD8.

Bone marrow is involved in about 20% of the cases. The involvement is often subtle and appears as small aggregate(s) of atypical lymphocytes with characteristic nuclear convolution. Diffuse marrow involvement is infrequent.

Clinical Aspects

Sézary syndrome/mycosis fungoides is a relatively uncommon disorder with predilection for older individuals (usually >50 years) and African Americans. The male:female ratio is about 2:1. In 10% to 15% of the patients, the disorder may transform to a large cell lymphoma.

Differential Diagnosis

Differential diagnosis of Sézary syndrome includes ATLL (see above) and a broad spectrum of chronic dermatitides, such as parapsoriasis and lichen planus. In these reactive conditions, lymphocytosis is polyclonal, with a mixture of CD4 and CD8 positive cells.

Selected References

Barcos M: Mycosis fungoides: Diagnosis and pathogenesis. Am J Clin Pathol 99:452, 1993.

Batata A, Shen B: Immunophenotyping of subtypes of B-chronic (mature) lymphoid leukemia. A study of 242 cases. Cancer 70:2436, 1992.

Bennett JM, Catovsky D, Daniel MT, et al: Proposals for the classification of chronic (mature) B and T lymphoid leukemias. J Clin Pathol 42:567, 1989.

Brunning RD: T-prolymphocytic leukemia. Blood 78:3111, 1991.

Chang KL, Stroup R, Weiss LM: Hairy cell leukemia: Current status. Am J Clin Pathol 97:719, 1992.

Cheson BD, Bennett JM, Grever M, et al: National Cancer Institute–Sponsored Working Group guidelines for chronic lymphocytic leukemia: Revised guidelines for diagnosis and treatment. Blood 87:4990, 1996.

Criel A, Michaux L, De Wolf-Peeters C: The concept of typical and atypical chronic lymphocytic leukaemia. Leuk Lymphoma 33:33, 1999.

Diamandidou E, Cohen PR, Kurzrock R: Mycosis fungoides and Sézary syndrome. Blood 88:2385, 1996.

Flinn IW, Grever MR: Chronic lymphocytic leukemia. Cancer Treat Rev 22:1, 1992.

Hamblin TJ, Oscier DG: Chronic lymphocytic leukemia: The nature of the leukemic cell. Blood Rev 11:229, 1997.

Hoyer JD, Ross CW, Li CY, et al: True T-cell chronic lymphocytic leukemia: A morphologic and immunophenotypic study of 25 cases. Blood 86:1163, 1995.

Kim YH, Hoppe RT: Mycosis fungoides and the Sézary syndrome. Semin Oncol 26:276, 1999.

Loughran TP: Clonal disease of large granular lymphocytes. Blood 82:1, 1993.

Melo JV, Catovsky D, Galton DAG: The relationship between chronic lymphocytic leukemia and prolymphocytic leukemia. 1. Clinical and laboratory features of 300 patients and characterization of an intermediate group. Br J Haematol 63:377, 1986.

Montserrat E, Villamor N, Reverter J-C, et al: Bone marrow assessment in B-cell chronic lymphocytic leukemia: Aspirate or biopsy? A comparative study in 258 patients. Brit J Haematol 93:111, 1996.

Oscier D: Chronic lymphocytic leukaemia. Br J Haematol 105(Suppl 1):1, 1999.

Robbins BA, Ellison DJ, Spinosa JC, et al: Diagnostic application of two-color flow cytometry in 161 cases of hairy cell leukemia. Blood 82:1277, 1993.

Robertson LE, Pugh W, O'Brien S, et al: Richter's syndrome: A report of 39 cases. J Clin Oncol 11:1985, 1993.

Scott CS, Richards SJ: Classification of large granular lymphocyte (LGL) and NK-associated disorders. Blood Rev 6:220, 1992.

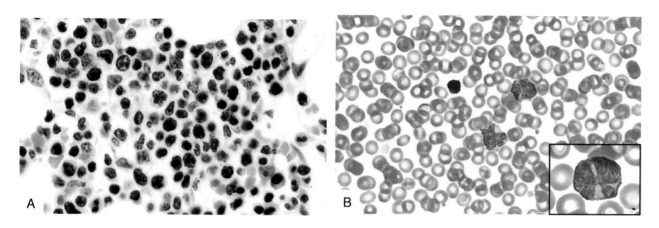

Figure 8–32. Adult T-cell leukemia/lymphoma. Bone marrow biopsy section (*A*), and blood smear (*B*) demonstrate increased numbers of atypical lymphocytes with irregular or convoluted nuclei. The inset shows a cell with marked nuclear convolution ("clover leaf" cell).

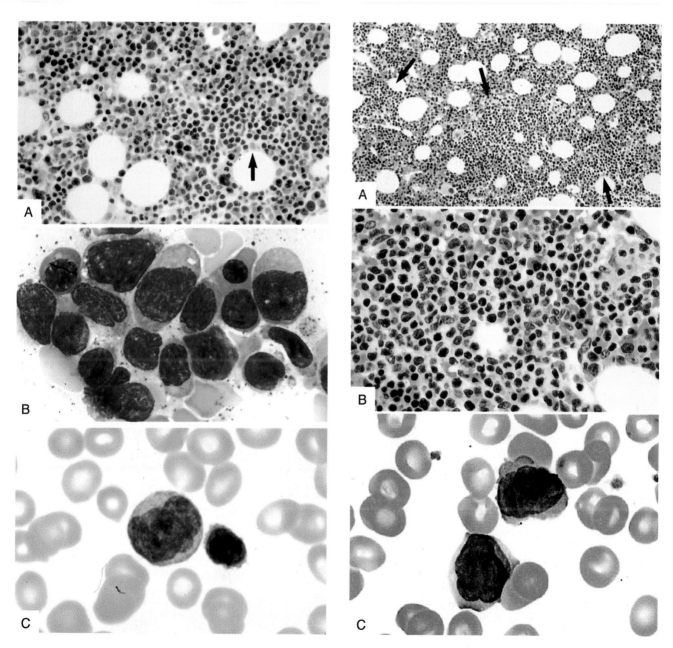

Figure 8–33. Sézary syndrome. Bone marrow biopsy section (*A, arrow*), bone marrow smear (*B*), and blood smear (*C*) demonstrate increased numbers of atypical lymphocytes with irregular or convoluted nuclei.

Figure 8–34. Sézary syndrome. Bone marrow biopsy section demonstrating aggregates of atypical lymphocytes with irregular or convoluted nuclei (*A, arrows,* and *B*). Blood smear demonstrating increased numbers of atypical lymphocytes with convoluted nuclei (*C*).

117

CHAPTER 9

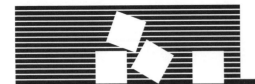

Malignant Lymphomas

Malignant lymphomas are the neoplasm of lymphoid cells arising in solid tissues. Lymph nodes are the most frequent primary site for lymphomas, but other organs such as skin, gastrointestinal tract, respiratory system, spleen, bone marrow, and central nervous system may also be the primary site. There is a significant overlap between lymphoid leukemias and malignant lymphomas; lymphoid leukemias often invade lymphoid tissues, and malignant lymphomas may infiltrate bone marrow and eventually involve peripheral blood. In some instances, such as in chronic lymphoid leukemia (CLL) and small lymphocytic lymphoma, leukemic or lymphomatous presentations are different clinical manifestations of the same disorder.

Bone marrow involvement in malignant lymphoma is often focal or patchy, and therefore the involved areas may be missed if the bone marrow samples are inadequate.

The pathologic features of malignant lymphomas are well presented in the *Atlas of Lymphoid Hyperplasia and Lymphoma*, by Ferry and Harris, in the Atlas in Diagnostic Surgical Pathology series (WB Saunders). Therefore, this chapter is brief and primarily provides representative examples of bone marrow involvement in malignant lymphomas.

CLASSIFICATION

Malignant lymphomas are divided into two major groups: Hodgkin's lymphoma (Hodgkin's disease) and non-Hodgkin's lymphoma (NHL). The bone marrow involvement is less frequent in Hodgkin's lymphoma than in non-Hodgkin's lymphomas.

Hodgkin's Lymphoma (Hodgkin's Disease)

Hodgkin's lymphoma (HL) is characterized by the presence of Reed-Sternberg (RS) cells in a background of inflammatory cells. The diagnostic ("classic") RS cell is a large binucleated cell with prominent round nucleoli and perinucleolar halos, displaying an "owl-eye" appearance (Figure 9–1). RS variants are large atypical mononuclear or multinuclear cells (Hodgkin's cells) that may display particular morphologic features in certain subclasses of HL, such as "popcorn" cells in lymphocyte-predominant

HL and "lacunar" cells in mixed-cellularity HL (Figures 9–2 and 9–3). The origin of RS cells and RS variants is still controversial, but recent investigations indicate a lymphoid origin, predominantly of B-cell lineage. The RS cells and their variants are intermixed with lymphocytes, plasma cells, eosinophils, histiocytes, and fibroblasts.

In the recently proposed classification by the World Health Organization (WHO), HL is divided into two major categories: nodular lymphocyte-predominant HL, and classical HL (Table 9–1). The classical HL includes nodular sclerosis, mixed-cellularity, and lymphocyte-depletion subtypes.

Nodular Lymphocyte-Predominant Hodgkin's Lymphoma

Lymphocyte-predominant Hodgkin's lymphoma (LPHL) is characterized by the presence of numerous mature lymphocytes, paucity of the diagnostic RS cells, and the presence of RS variants known as "popcorn" cells. Popcorn cells are large cells with scant to moderate amounts of cytoplasm; a large, delicate, multilobated nucleus; and multiple small nucleoli (see Figure 9–2). They express CD45 and B cell–associated antigens (CD19, CD20, CD22, CD79a) and are negative for CD15, CD30, and Epstein-Barr virus (EBV). The pattern of lymph node involvement is nodular with or without diffuse areas, and some lesions may show large numbers of histiocytes. LPHL appears to represent a polyclonal B-cell lymphoproliferative process that may eventually progress to a monoclonal disorder, which is often a large B-cell lymphoma. LPHL usually does not involve bone marrow.

Classical Hodgkin's Lymphoma

Classical HL is defined by the presence of diagnostic (classic) RS cells and their variants. These cells often express CD15 and CD30+ and are negative for CD45 (Figure 9–4). In approximately 5% to 20% of the cases of HL, RS cells and variants may express CD20, but they are usually negative for B and T cell–associated antigens.

Nodular sclerosis HL (NSHL) is characterized by the presence of lacunar cells (RS cell variant) and nodular compartmentalization of the involved lymph node by collagen (Figure 9–5). Lacunar cells are large cells with abundant pale cytoplasm, a large lobulated nucleus, and

118

small nucleoli. These cells in the formalin–fixed tissue preparations, due to the retraction of the cytoplasm caused by the fixation process, appear to be sitting in an empty space (lacuna) (see Figures 9–2 and 9–5). In 15% to 30% of the cases of NSHL, RS cells and variants show evidence of EBV infection. Bone marrow is involved in about 5% of the cases.

Mixed-cellularity HL (MCHL) displays numerous classic RS cells and RS variants. The pattern of involvement is diffuse or vaguely nodular without band-forming sclerosis. The infiltrate contains lymphocytes, plasma cells, histiocytes, eosinophils, and neutrophils. In 60% to 70% of the cases of MCHL, RS cells and variants show evidence of EBV infection. Bone marrow is involved in about 5% of the cases (Figures 9–6 and 9–7).

Lymphocyte-depletion HL (LDHL) is characterized by a diffuse infiltrate that is often associated with diffuse fibrosis, areas of necrosis, and paucity of other inflammatory cells (Figures 9–8 and 9–9). RS cells and bizarre RS variants are present. Bone marrow involvement is frequent.

Clinical Aspects

Four clinical stages are defined for HL and NHL. Stage 1 is defined as the involvement of one lymph node region or a single extranodal tissue. Stage II is involvement of two lymph node regions on the same side of the diaphragm, with or without involvement of limited contiguous extranodal tissues. Stage III involves lymph nodes on both sides of the diaphragm, with or without involvement of the spleen and/or limited contiguous extranodal tissues, and Stage IV refers to disseminated or multiple foci of involvement of one or more extranodal tissues. All the stages are divided into A or B on the basis of the presence or absence of systemic symptoms (fever, weight loss, night sweats), respectively. Most of the patients with LPHL and NSHL have localized disease.

Most frequent sites of lymphadenopathy are in the axillary and inguinal areas (about 70%), followed by mediastinal (around 60%) and retroperitoneal (about 25%) regions. Mediastinal involvement is one of the characteristic features of NSHL, and retroperitoneal involvement is more frequently seen in LDHL. The frequency of extranodal involvement (such as bone marrow, gastrointestinal tract, central nervous system, and skin) is significantly less in HL than in NHL.

Differential Diagnosis

Differential diagnosis includes bone marrow lesions with histiocytic components (granulomas, Langerhans cell histiocytosis), disorders that are associated with marrow fibrosis with trapped megakaryocytes (myelofibrosis), and metastatic tumor cells that mimic RS cells. LPHL is distinguished from low-grade B-cell lymphomas by the presence of the popcorn cells (positive for CD45 and B-cell markers and negative for CD15 and CD30). The lymphocytes are a mixture of B and T cells, and the B-cell component is often polyclonal. Anaplastic large cell lymphoma may contain cells that are similar to RS cells or RS variants. These cells are CD30 positive, but also express CD45. Megakaryocytes may morphologically mimic RS cells, but they express factor VIII and are negative for CD15 and CD30 antigens.

Non-Hodgkin's Lymphomas

Bone marrow is a frequent site of involvement in patients with non-Hodgkin's lymphoma (NHL). However, primary involvement of bone (or bone marrow) with NHL is rare. The topography of bone marrow involvement in NHL is diverse and includes focal, nodular (patchy), paratrabecular, interstitial, diffuse, or a combination of these patterns.

In a significant proportion of lymphomas (ranging from 15% to 70% in various reports), bone marrow involvement is morphologically different from the lymph node involvement in the same patient. This morphologic discordance may sometimes create diagnostic and classification problems. Frequently, lymphoma in the involved

Table 9–1
THE PROPOSED WHO CLASSIFICATION OF LYMPHOID NEOPLASMS*

B-CELL NEOPLASMS
Precursor B-cell lymphoblastic leukemia/lymphoma
Mature B-cell neoplasms
  B-cell chronic lymphocytic leukemia/small lymphocytic lymphoma
  B-cell prolymphocytic leukemia
  Lymphoplasmacytic lymphoma
  Mantle cell lymphoma
  Follicular lymphoma
  Marginal zone B-cell lymphoma of mucosa-associated lymphoid tissue (MALT) type
  Nodal marginal zone lymphoma
  Splenic marginal zone B-cell lymphoma
  Hairy cell leukemia
  Diffuse large B-cell lymphoma (including mediastinal, intravascular, and primary effusion types)
  Burkitt's lymphoma/leukemia
  Plasma cell myeloma/plasmacytoma

T-CELL NEOPLASMS
Precursor T-cell lymphoblastic leukemia/lymphoma
Mature T-cell and NK-cell neoplasms
  T-cell prolymphocytic leukemia
  T-cell large granular lymphocytic leukemia
  Aggressive NK-cell leukemia
  T-NK–cell lymphoma, nasal and nasal-type (angiocentric lymphoma)
  Mycosis fungoides and Sézary syndrome
  Angioimmunoblastic T-cell lymphoma
  Peripheral T-cell lymphomas
  Adult T-cell leukemia/lymphoma (HTLV1+)
  Anaplastic large cell lymphoma
  Primary cutaneous CD30+ T-cell lymphoproliferative disorders
  Subcutaneous panniculitis-like T-cell lymphoma
  Entropathy-type intestinal T-cell lymphoma
  Hepatosplenic γ/δ T-cell lymphoma

HODGKIN'S LYMPHOMA (HODGKIN'S DISEASE)
Nodular lymphocyte-predominant (Hodgkin's lymphoma)
Classical Hodgkin's lymphoma
  Nodular sclerosis
  Mixed cellularity
  Lymphocyte depletion

* Adapted from Harris NL, et al: Mod Pathol 13:193, 2000.
  WHO = World Health Organization; HTLV = human T-cell lymphotrophic virus; NK = natural killer.

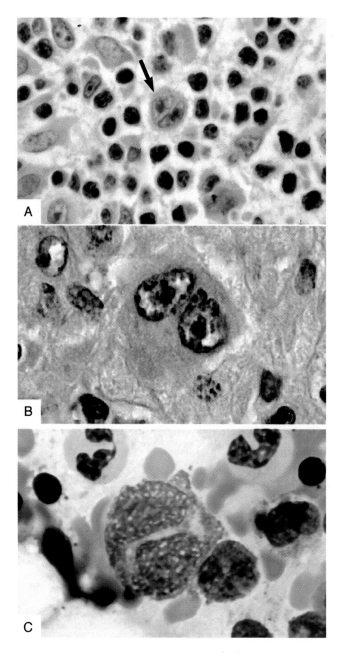

Figure 9-1. Classic Reed-Sternberg cells are large, binucleated cells with prominent round nucleoli and perinucleolar halos, displaying an "owl-eye" appearance; bone marrow biopsy sections (*A* and *B*) and marrow smear (*C*).

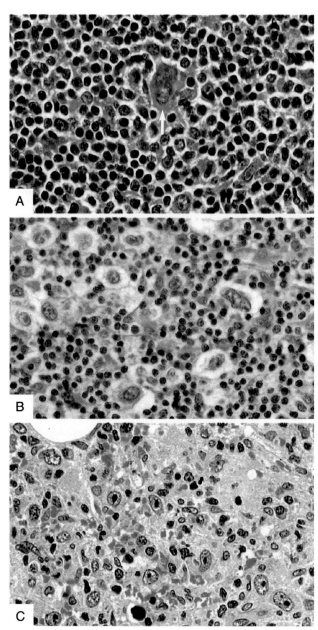

Figure 9-2. Reed-Sternberg (RS) variants are large atypical mononuclear or multinuclear cells that may display particular morphologic features in certain subclasses of Hodgkin's lymphoma (HL). *A* demonstrates a "popcorn" cell in lymphocyte predominant HL (*arrow*), *B* shows "lacunar" cells in mixed-cellularity HL, and *C* displays numerous large mononuclear RS variants in a case of lymphocyte-depletion HL.

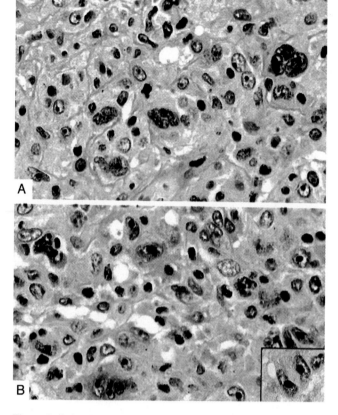

Figure 9–3. Reed-Sternberg (RS) variants. Numerous large, multinucleated cells or cells with multilobular nuclei are demonstrated in lymph node biopsy section of a patient with lymphocyte-depletion HL. The inset shows a classic RS cell.

bone marrow appears less aggressive than that in the lymph node. Because of this discordant morphology, it is highly recommended that the classification of lymphoma be based on the evaluation of the involved lymph node and not the bone marrow.

The classification of NHL has gone through several cycles of revisions and modifications. The currently popular classification proposed by the International Lymphoma Study Group, known as the Revised European-American Lymphoma (REAL) classification, has been recently challenged by a newly proposed classification by WHO (see Table 9–1). However, the WHO classification is basically similar to the REAL classification with some minor modifications. Both the REAL and WHO classifications are classifications for lymphoid malignancies and therefore include lymphoid leukemias (chronic and acute) and plasma cell neoplasms. Lymphoid leukemias and plasma cell disorders are discussed in Chapters 6, 8, and 10. The common forms of NHLs are briefly discussed below.

Small Lymphocytic Lymphoma/CLL

Morphologic features of bone marrow involvement are discussed in Chapter 8 (see Figures 8–1 to 8–6 and 9–10). The involved lymph nodes show diffuse infiltration of mature, small lymphocytes with scanty blue cytoplasm, round to slightly irregular nucleus, and dense

chromatin. One of the characteristic morphologic features is the presence of pale areas of proliferation centers (pseudofollicles) consisting of prolymphocytes and para-immunoblasts (Figure 9–10).

Small lymphocytic lymphoma is a B-cell malignancy. The major immunophenotypic features of the tumor cells include expression of CD5, CD23, CD19, CD20, and CD43 and lack of expression of CD10. Trisomy 12 and abnormalities of 13q and del(6q) are the most frequent cytogenetic abnormalities.

Lymphoplasmacytic Lymphoma

Lymphoplasmacytic lymphoma consists of small B lymphocytes, plasmacytoid lymphocytes, and plasma cells (Figures 9–11 to 9–13). The tumor cells are negative for CD5 and CD10, but usually express other B cell–associated antigens. Lymphoplasmacytic lymphoma is often associated with Waldenström's macroglobulinemia (see Chapter 10), and frequently (up to 50%) shows t(9;14) translocation.

Mantle Cell Lymphoma

Mantle cell lymphoma is characterized by proliferation of small to intermediate-sized mature B lymphocytes. The nuclear morphology varies from round to cleaved, with clumped to dispersed chromatin (Figures 9–14 and 9–15). The blastic mantle cell lymphoma is composed of either lymphoblast-like cells with inconspicuous nucleoli or large pleomorphic cells with prominent nucleoli (Figure 9–16). The neoplastic cells express CD5, CD19, CD20, and CD79a, are cyclin D1 (bcl-1) positive, and lack CD10 and CD23. The characteristic cytogenetic feature of the mantle cell lymphoma is t(11;14) translocation.

Marginal Zone B-Cell Lymphoma

Marginal zone B-cell lymphoma is divided into nodal, mucosa-associated (MALT), and splenic subtypes. The nodal lesions and MALT lymphoma often demonstrate monocytoid features (monocytoid B cells), and the splenic variants display white pulp nodules with a central core of small lymphocytes surrounded by a pale rim of splenic marginal zone-type cells (Figure 9–17). The tumor cells in blood or bone marrow smears may show cytoplasmic projections resembling hairy cell leukemia (Figure 9–18). Bone marrow biopsy sections may demonstrate sinusoidal involvement (Figure 9–19). Most of the cases of lymphomas referred to as "splenic lymphoma with villous lymphocytes" fall into the category of splenic marginal zone lymphoma. The tumor cells express CD19, CD20, and CD22 and are usually negative for CD5, CD10, and CD23, as well as CD103 and TRAP. So far, no characteristic cytogenetic abnormalities have been reported.

Follicular Lymphoma

Follicular lymphoma is malignancy of the cleaved and noncleaved follicular center cells (Figures 9–20 and

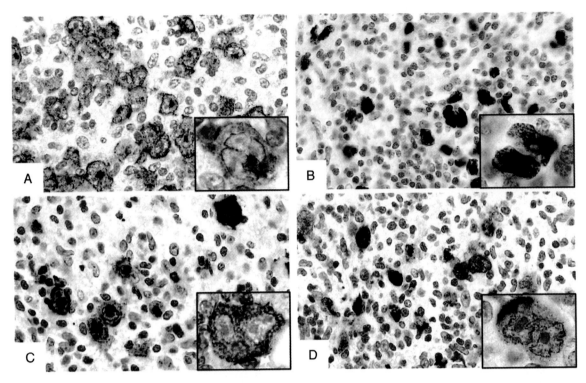

Figure 9–4. Hodgkin's lymphoma (HL). Lymph node biopsy sections demonstrate classic RS cells (insets) and RS variants expressing CD30 (*A*), EBV, EBER (*B*), CD15 (*C*) and EBV, LMP (*D*).

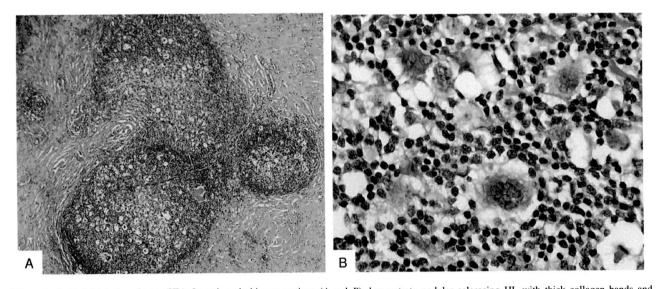

Figure 9–5. Hodgkin's lymphoma (HL). Lymph node biopsy sections (*A* and *B*) demonstrate nodular sclerosing HL with thick collagen bands and numerous lacunar cells.

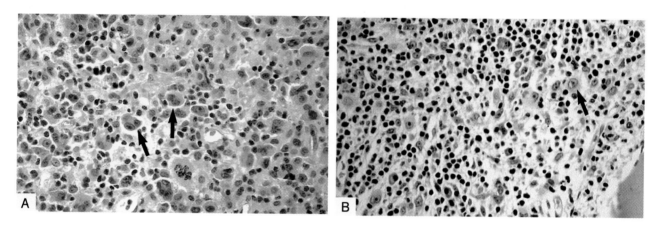

Figure 9–6. Hodgkin's lymphoma (HL). Bone marrow biopsy section demonstrating involvement with HL. Numerous RS variants are mixed with a lymphohistiocytic infiltrate (low-power [*A*] and high-power [*B*] views).

Figure 9–7. Hodgkin's lymphoma (HL). Lymph node biopsy section (*A*) demonstrates numerous classic RS cells (*arrows*) and RS variants representing a mixed-cellularity HL. Bone marrow biopsy section (*B*) shows focal involvement with scattered RS variant mixed with lymphocytes and fibroblasts.

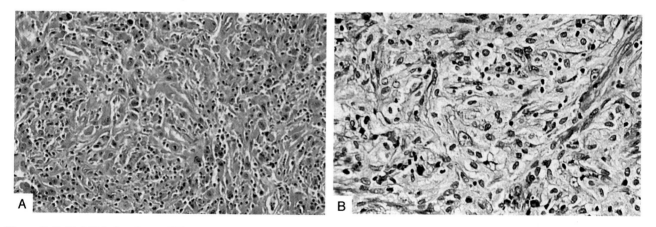

Figure 9–8. Hodgkin's lymphoma (HL). Lymph node biopsy sections demonstrate morphologic variants of lymphocyte depletion HL. *A*, With numerous RS variant, and *B*, with occasional RS variants. Both show extensive fibrosis.

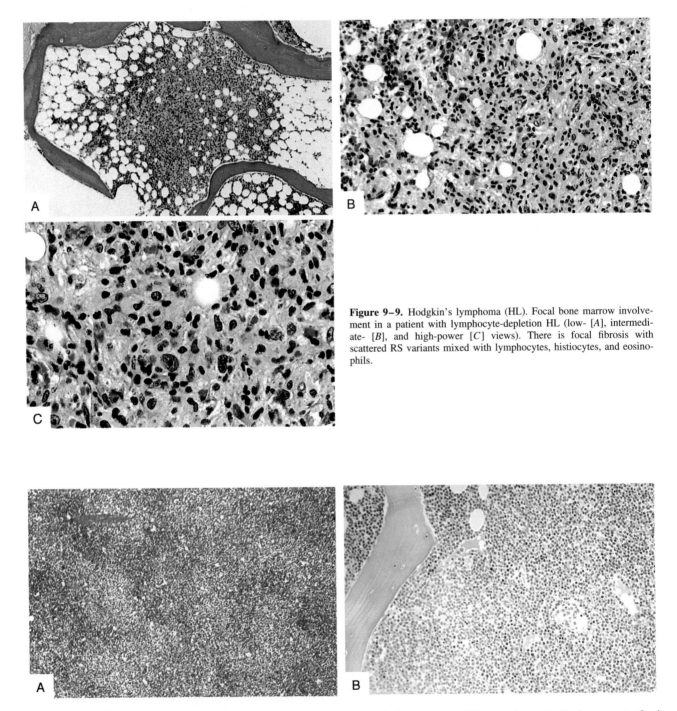

Figure 9–9. Hodgkin's lymphoma (HL). Focal bone marrow involvement in a patient with lymphocyte-depletion HL (low- [A], intermediate- [B], and high-power [C] views). There is focal fibrosis with scattered RS variants mixed with lymphocytes, histiocytes, and eosinophils.

Figure 9–10. Small lymphocytic lymphoma (SLL). Lymph node biopsy section (A) demonstrates a diffuse involvement with the presence of pale areas of proliferation centers (pseudofollicles). Bone marrow biopsy section (B) demonstrates a diffuse infiltration of small mature lymphocytes. SLL and CLL share similar clinicopathologic features (see Chapter 8, Figures 8–1 to 8–6).

9–21). Most cases consist of small and/or large cleaved cells with complete or partial preservation of the follicular structures. Bone marrow involvement is predominantly paratrabecular (see Figures 9–20 and 9–21). The tumor cells express CD19 and CD20, are often CD10-positive, and are CD5-negative. They also express bcl-2 and bcl-6 proteins. The characteristic cytogenetic feature of follicular lymphoma is t(14;18) translocation.

Diffuse Large Cell Lymphoma

Diffuse large cell lymphoma is characterized by a diffuse proliferation of the transformed large neoplastic lymphoid cells (Figures 9–22 to 9–24). The nuclei of the tumor cells are larger than the nuclei of normal histiocytes. The cytologic features of the neoplastic cells may vary from case to case. Several morphologic subtypes, such as immunoblastic, polymorphous, clear cell, and multilobulated forms have been reported. Bone marrow involvement in some cases may be obscured by the lack of a detectable lymphoid aggregate. However, careful examination of the bone marrow may reveal the presence of scattered tumor cells interspersed with normal marrow cells (see Figure 9–24). The neoplastic cells in the majority of the cases are of B-cell origin and express CD19, CD20, CD22, and CD79a. They may also demonstrate variable expression of activation antigens (such as CD25, CD30, and CD38). A small proportion of the cases may express CD5 and/or CD10. Frequent cytogenetic abnormalities include t(14;18) and t(3;14).

Burkitt's Lymphoma

Burkitt's lymphoma consists of a highly proliferative, relatively monomorphic neoplastic lymphoid blasts with scanty, often vacuolated cytoplasm, finely dispersed chromatin, and prominent nucleoli (Figure 9–25). The morphologic features and biologic behavior of Burkitt's lymphoma are similar to those of ALL-L3 (see Chapter 6). The tumor cells express membrane Ig and B cell–associated antigens (CD19, CD20, CD22, and CD79a), but are CD5- and CD23-negative, and may express CD10. Cytogenetic abnormalities include t(8;14), t(2;8), and t(8;22).

Peripheral T-Cell Lymphomas

This group includes a garden variety of post-thymic T-lymphoproliferative disorders with highly variable morphologic features. The neoplastic cells vary from small, cleaved cells to large pleomorphic cells, and are often admixed with inflammatory cells, particularly epithelioid histiocytes (Figure 9–26). Most cases of peripheral T-cell lymphomas are CD4-positive.

Anaplastic Large Cell Lymphoma

Anaplastic large cell lymphoma is characterized by the presence of large anaplastic lymphoid cells with abundant cytoplasm, large and pleomorphic nuclei, and prominent nucleoli (Figure 9–27). Multinuclated RS-like cells are often present. The tumor cells are usually of T-cell type, and express CD30 (Ki-1) and epithelial membrane antigens (EMA). Anaplastic large cell lymphoma has been associated with t(2;5) translocation (ALK/NPM genes), and expression of the ALK protein.

NK/T-Cell Lymphoma, Nasal and Nasal-Type

This group consists of highly aggressive and angioinvasive lymphomas (see Figure 9–27). The neoplastic cells display variable cytologic features and express CD2, CD8, and CD56. They are usually negative for membrane CD3, but often show cytoplasmic CD3. EBV is frequently positive.

Angioimmunoblastic T-Cell Lymphoma

Angioimmunoblastic T-cell lymphoma is a rare lymphoproliferative disorder characterized by diffuse infiltration of large atypical lymphoid cells and T-immunoblasts admixed with histiocytes and eosinophils. The large atypical cells have a tendency to appear in clusters, particularly around blood vessels.

Others

A plasmablastic variant of malignant lymphoma, associated with human herpes virus 8 (HHV-8), has been observed in some patients with AIDS (Figure 9–28) or Castleman disease. HHV-8 plays a role in pathogenesis of Kaposi's sarcoma and has been found in cells of primary effusion lymphomas.

Clinical Aspects

Clinical staging and pathologic classifications are major prognostic indicators in NHL. Several other parameters have been correlated with the prognosis. For example, elevated S-phase fraction of the cell cycle and overexpression of Ki-67 (a proliferation-associated antigen) have been associated with poor prognosis. Classification and clinical behavior of the NHLs are correlated in Table 9–2.

Differential Diagnosis

There is some morphologic overlap between low- and intermediate-grade NHLs, particularly those with mature, small or medium-size lymphocytes, such as small lymphocytic; mantle cell; marginal zone; and small, cleaved follicular lymphomas. However, these subtypes often have distinct immunophenotypic and cytogenetic/DNA molecular features. It is sometimes difficult to distinguish LDHL from anaplastic large cell lymphoma. The leukemic phase of marginal zone lymphoma may mimic hairy cell leukemia (HCL). HCL cells are TRAP-positive and usually express CD103, whereas marginal cells are TRAP-negative and infrequently express CD103. Reactive lymphoid aggregates, histiocytic lesions (such as granulomas and Langerhans's cell histiocytosis), increased hematogones in regenerating bone marrows, metastatic round cell tumors, metastatic melanoma, and mast cell disorders may mimic NHLs. Bone marrow sections from patients treated for B-cell NHL may show atypical aggregates of reactive T cells that morphologically resemble residual lymphoma (Figure 9–29).

Selected References

Brunning RD, McKenna RW: Atlas of Tumors of the Bone Marrow. Washington, DC, Armed Forces Institute of Pathology, 1994, p 360.

Brunning RD, McKenna RW: Bone marrow manifestations of malignant lymphoma and lymphoma-like conditions. Pathol Ann 14:1, 1979.

Butler JJ, Pugh WC: Review of Hodgkin's disease. Hematol Pathol 7:59, 1993.

Campo E, Raffeld M, Jaffe ES: Mantle-cell lymphoma. Semin Hematol 36:115, 1999.

Catovsky D, Matutes E: Splenic lymphoma with circulating villous lymphocytes/splenic marginal-zone lymphoma. Semin Hematol 36:148, 1999.

Conlan MG, Bast M, Armitage JO, et al: Bone marrow involvement by non-Hodgkin's lymphoma: The clinical significance of morphologic discordance between the lymph node and bone marrow. Nebraska Lymphoma Study Group. J Clin Oncol 8:1163, 1990.

Douglas VK, Gordon LI, Goolsby CL, et al: Lymphoid aggregates in bone marrow mimic residual lymphoma after therapy for non-Hodgkin lymphoma. Am J Clin Pathol 112:844, 1999.

Duplin N, Diss TL, Kellam P, et al: HHV-8 is associated with plasmablastic variant of Castleman disease that is linked to HHV-8–positive plasmablastic lymphoma. Blood 95:1406, 2000.

Falini B, Pileri S, Zinzani PL, et al: ALK+ lymphoma: Clinico-pathological findings and outcome. Blood 93:2697, 1999.

Fraga M, Brosset P, Schaifer D, et al: Bone marrow involvement in anaplastic large cell lymphoma. Immunohistochemical detection of minimal disease and its prognostic significance. Am J Clin Pathol 103:82, 1995.

Ghani AM, Krause JR: Bone marrow biopsy findings in angioimmunoblastic lymphadenopathy. Br J Haematol 61:203, 1985.

Harris NL: Hodgkin's disease: Classification and differential diagnosis. Mod Pathol 12:159, 1999.

Harris NL, Jaffe ES, Diebold J, et al: The World Health Organization classification of hematological malignancies. Report of the Clinical Advisory Committee Meeting. Airlie House, Virginia, November 1997. Mod Pathol 13:193, 2000.

Harris NL, Jaffe ES, Stein H, et al: A revised European-American classification of lymphoid neoplasms: A proposal from the International Lymphoma Study Group. Blood 84:1361, 1994.

Hodges GF, Lenherdt TM, Coteligam JD: Bone marrow involvement in large-cell lymphoma. Prognostic implications of discordant disease. Am J Clin Pathol 101:305, 1994.

Isaacson PG, Matutes E, Burke M, et al: The histopathology of splenic lymphoma with villous lymphocytes. Blood 84:3828, 1994.

Jaffe ES, Harris NL, Diebold J, et al: World Health Organization classification of neoplastic diseases of the hematopoietic and lymphoid tissues. Am J Clin Pathol 111:S8, 1999.

Juneja SK, Wolf MM, Cooper IA: Value of bilateral bone marrow biopsy specimens in non-Hodgkin's lymphoma. J Clin Pathol 43:630, 1990.

Labourie E, Marit G, Vial J, et al: Intrasinusoidal bone marrow involvement by splenic lymphoma with villous lymphocytes: A helpful immunohistochemical feature. Mod Pathol 10:1015, 1997.

Macon WR, Williams ME, Greer JP, et al: Natural killer-like T-cell lymphomas: Aggressive lymphomas of T-large granular lymphocytes. Blood 87:1483, 1996.

Nathwani BN, Drachenberg MR, Hernandez AM, et al: Nodal monocytoid B-cell lymphoma (nodal marginal-zone B-cell lymphoma). Semin Hematol 36:128, 1999.

Pangalis GA, Angelopoulou MK, Vassilakopoulos TP, et al: B-chronic lymphocytic leukemia, small lymphocytic lymphoma, and lymphoplasmacytic lymphoma, including Waldenström's macroglobulinemia: A clinical, morphologic, and biologic spectrum of similar disorders. Semin Hematol 36:104, 1999.

Shin SS, Sheibani K: Monocytoid B cell lymphoma. Am J Clin Pathol 99:421, 1993.

Stein HS, Hummel M: Hodgkin's disease: Biology and origin of Hodgkin and Reed-Sternberg cells. Cancer Treat Rev 25:161, 1999.

Wasman J, Rosenthal NS, Farhi DC: Mantle cell lymphoma; morphologic findings in bone marrow involvement. Am J Clin Pathol 106:196, 1996.

Wu CD, Jackson CL, Medeiros J: Splenic marginal zone cell lymphoma; an immunophenotypic and molecular study of five cases. Am J Clin Pathol 105:277, 1996.

Zukerberg L, Medeiros L, Ferry J, et al: Diffuse low-grade B cell lymphomas: Four clinically distinct subtypes defined by a combination of morphologic and immunophenotypic features. Am J Clin Pathol 100:373, 1993.

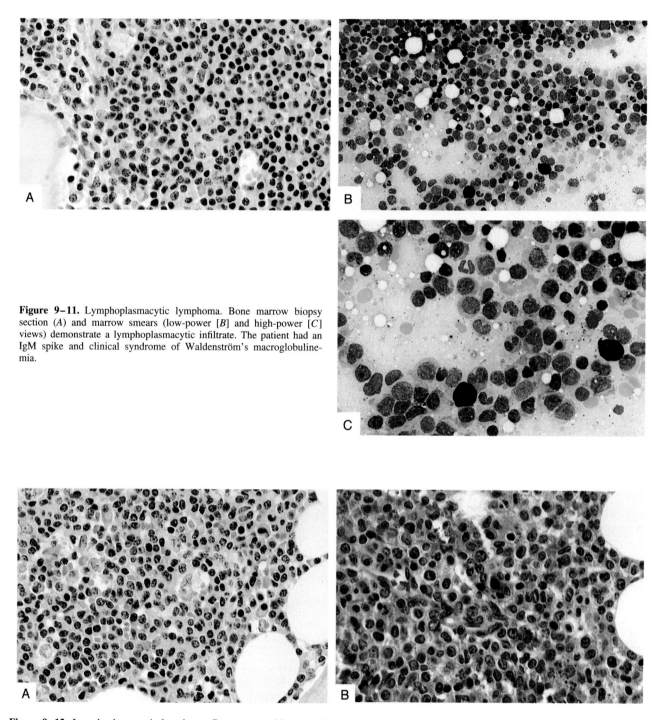

Figure 9–11. Lymphoplasmacytic lymphoma. Bone marrow biopsy section (*A*) and marrow smears (low-power [*B*] and high-power [*C*] views) demonstrate a lymphoplasmacytic infiltrate. The patient had an IgM spike and clinical syndrome of Waldenström's macroglobulinemia.

Figure 9–12. Lymphoplasmacytic lymphoma. Bone marrow biopsy sections (*A* and *B*) demonstrate a lymphoplasmacytic infiltrate. Iron particles are stained blue (*B*).

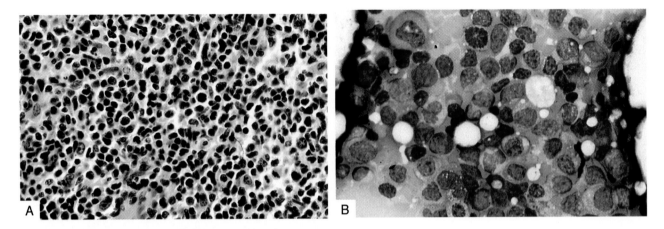

Figure 9–13. Lymphoplasmacytic lymphoma. Bone marrow biopsy section (*A*) and marrow smear (*B*) demonstrate an atypical lymphoplasmacytic infiltrate in a patient with Waldenström's macroglobulinemia (IgM spike).

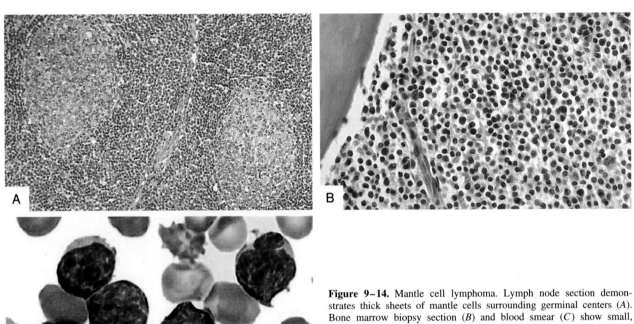

Figure 9–14. Mantle cell lymphoma. Lymph node section demonstrates thick sheets of mantle cells surrounding germinal centers (*A*). Bone marrow biopsy section (*B*) and blood smear (*C*) show small, mature lymphocytes with round or irregular nuclei.

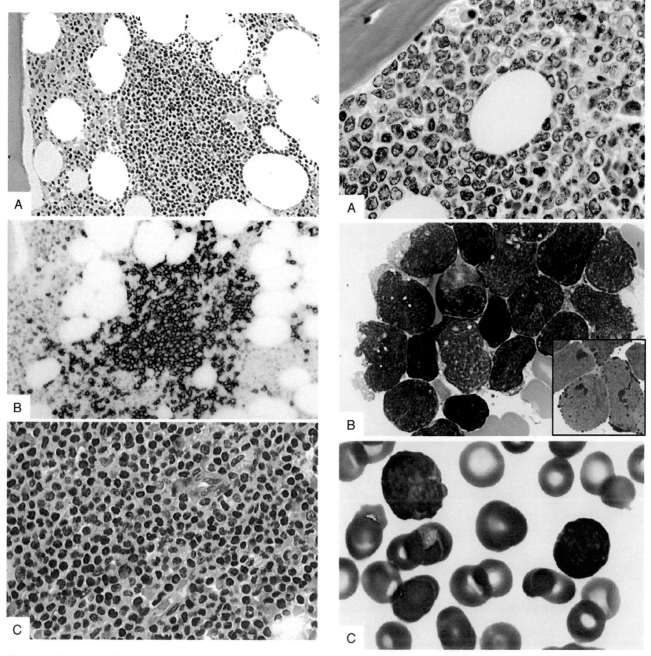

Figure 9–15. Mantle cell lymphoma. A lymphoid aggregate consisting of small, mature lymphocytes is demonstrated in the bone marrow biopsy section of a patient with mantle cell lymphoma (*A*). Lymphoid cells expressed CD20 (*B*) as well as CD5 and BCL-1 and were CD23-negative (data not shown). Higher power view of the bone marrow biopsy demonstrates small, mature lymphocytes with irregular nuclei (*C*).

Figure 9–16. Mantle cell lymphoma, blastic type. Bone marrow biopsy section (*A*), and bone marrow (*B*) and blood (*C*) smears demonstrate the presence of immature blast-like cells with scanty cytoplasm, irregular nuclei, and finely dispersed nuclear chromatin. The inset shows coarse periodic acid-Schiff (PAS)-positive cytoplasmic granules in the tumor cells. These cells expressed CD5, CD20, BCL-1, and Ig kappa light chain and were negative for CD23 (data not shown).

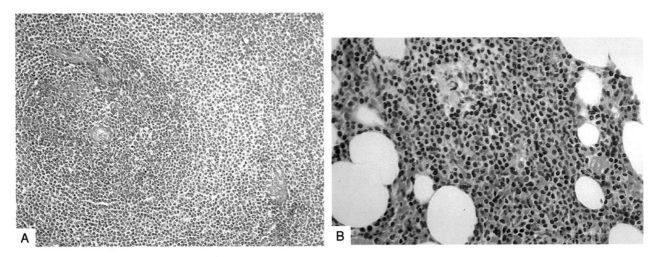

Figure 9–17. Marginal zone B-cell lymphoma. Spleen section demonstrates the expansion of marginal zone with increased numbers of medium-size lymphocytes (*A*). Bone marrow biopsy section shows an atypical aggregate of lymphocytes with nuclear spacing and irregularity (*B*). (From Naeim F: Pathology of Bone Marrow, 2nd ed. Baltimore, Williams & Wilkins, 1998, with permission.)

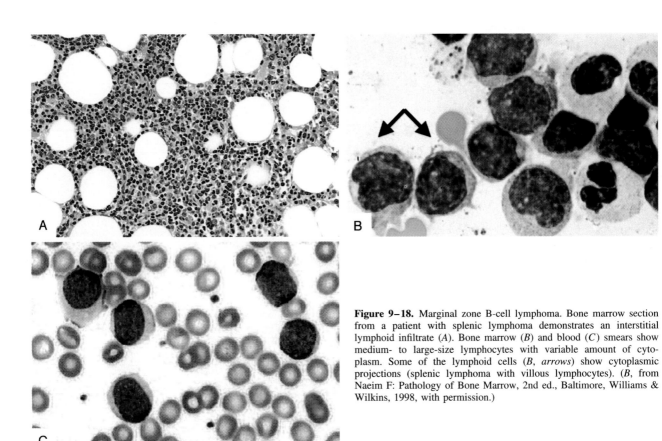

Figure 9–18. Marginal zone B-cell lymphoma. Bone marrow section from a patient with splenic lymphoma demonstrates an interstitial lymphoid infiltrate (*A*). Bone marrow (*B*) and blood (*C*) smears show medium- to large-size lymphocytes with variable amount of cytoplasm. Some of the lymphoid cells (*B*, *arrows*) show cytoplasmic projections (splenic lymphoma with villous lymphocytes). (*B*, from Naeim F: Pathology of Bone Marrow, 2nd ed., Baltimore, Williams & Wilkins, 1998, with permission.)

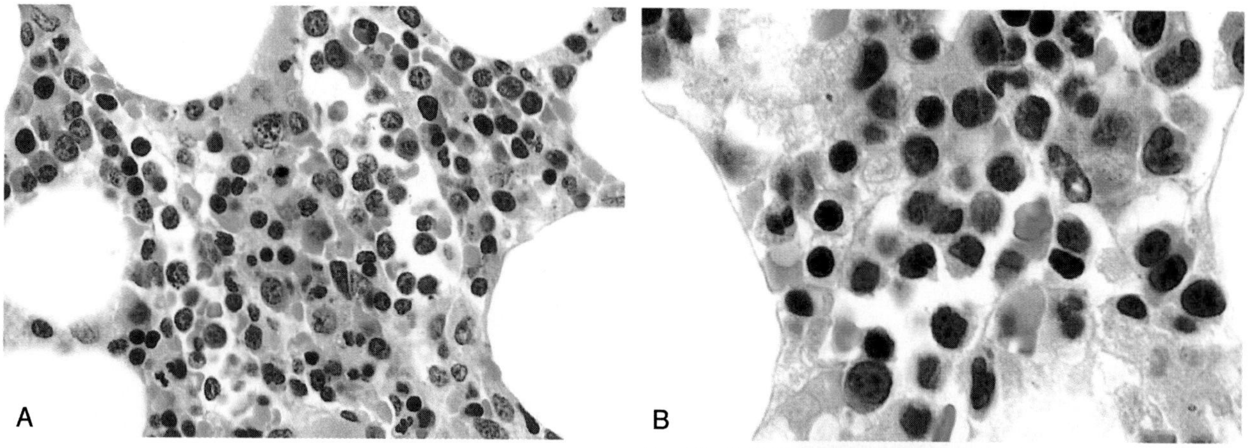

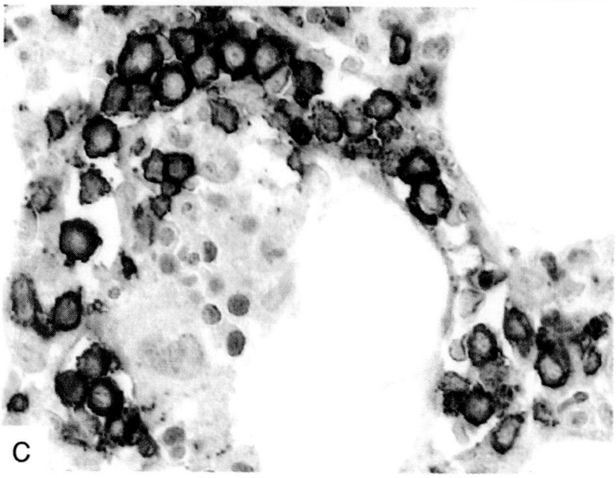

Figure 9–19. Marginal zone B-cell lymphoma. Biopsy section (low-power [A] and high-power [B] views) demonstrate sinusoidal infiltration by the tumor cells. Immunohistochemical stain for CD20 shows clusters of positive cells within the sinusoids (C).

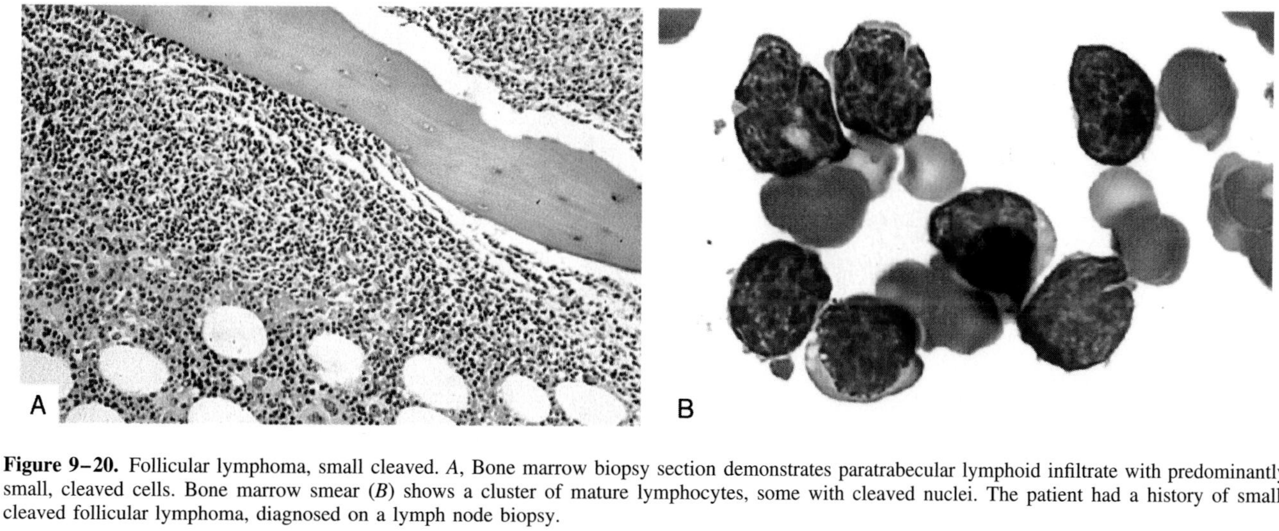

Figure 9–20. Follicular lymphoma, small cleaved. A, Bone marrow biopsy section demonstrates paratrabecular lymphoid infiltrate with predominantly small, cleaved cells. Bone marrow smear (B) shows a cluster of mature lymphocytes, some with cleaved nuclei. The patient had a history of small, cleaved follicular lymphoma, diagnosed on a lymph node biopsy.

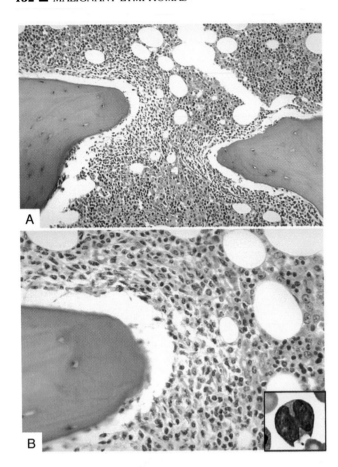

Figure 9–21. Follicular lymphoma, small cleaved. Bone marrow biopsy section (low-power [A] and high-power [B] views) from a patient with small, cleaved follicular lymphoma demonstrates paratrabecular lymphoid infiltrate with predominantly small, cleaved cells. Blood smear (inset) shows a mature lymphocyte with cleaved nucleus.

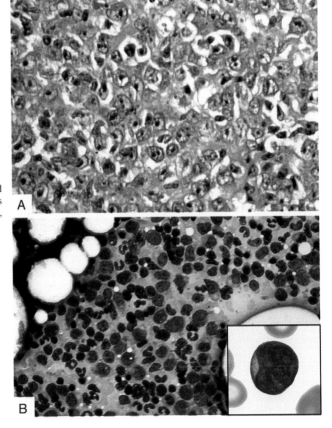

Figure 9–22. Large cell lymphoma. Bone marrow biopsy section (A) and marrow smear (B) demonstrate sheets of large, immature lymphoid cells with a variable amount of cytoplasm, finely dispersed nuclear chromatin, and prominent nucleoli. The inset shows a large blast cell (blood smear).

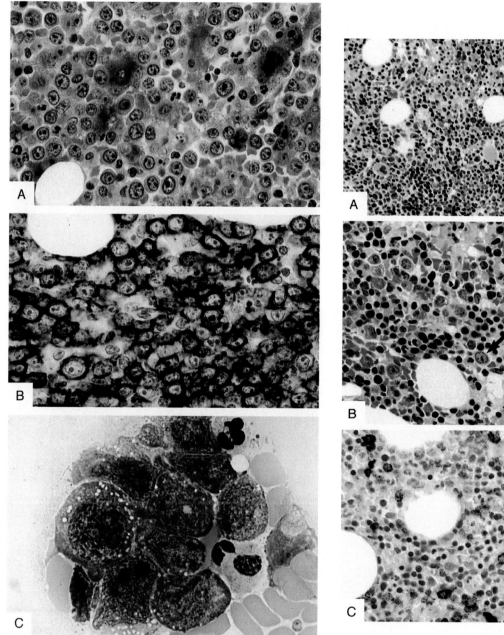

Figure 9-23. Large cell lymphoma. Bone marrow biopsy section (*A*) demonstrates sheets of large immature lymphoid cells with a variable amount of cytoplasm, finely dispersed nuclear chromatin, and prominent nucleoli (H & E and iron stains). The tumor cells (*B*) strongly express CD20 (immunoperoxidase stain). Bone marrow smear (*C*) shows a cluster of large, immature cells with dark, vacuolated, blue cytoplasm and round or slightly irregular nuclei. These cells resemble early megaloblastic erythroid precursors, such as rubriblasts and prorubricytes.

Figure 9-24. Large cell lymphoma. Bone marrow biopsy section from a patient with a history of B-large cell lymphoma demonstrates no evidence of lymphoid aggregates (low-power [*A*] and high-power [*B*] views). However, scattered large immature cells are present (*B*), some of which express CD20 (*C*, immunoperoxidase stain). The findings are consistent with bone marrow involvement.

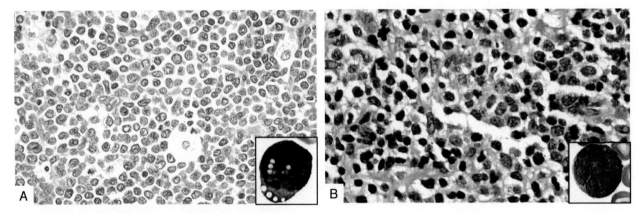

Figure 9–25. Burkitt's leukemia/lymphoma. Lymph node biopsy section (*A*) demonstrates sheets of monomorphic blasts and scattered macrophages (starry sky pattern). The inset shows a circulating blast cell with vacuolated cytoplasm. For comparison, *B* represents a lymph node section from a patient with precursor T-lymphoblastic leukemia/lymphoma. Blast cells show irregular nuclei, fine nuclear chromatin, and inconspicuous nucleoli. The inset demonstrates a circulating blast.

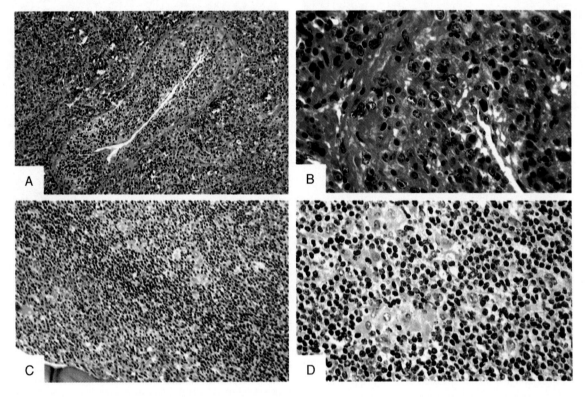

Figure 9–26. Peripheral T-cell lymphomas. Biopsy section from a mediastinal mass displaying an angioinvasive tumor (low-power [*A*] and high-power [*B*] views). The tumor cells expressed CD3, CD8, and CD56 (data not shown). Bone marrow biopsy section from a patient with history of T-cell lymphoma (Lennert's type) demonstrating sheets of lymphocytes and aggregates of epithelioid histiocytes (low-power [*C*] and high-power [*D*] views).

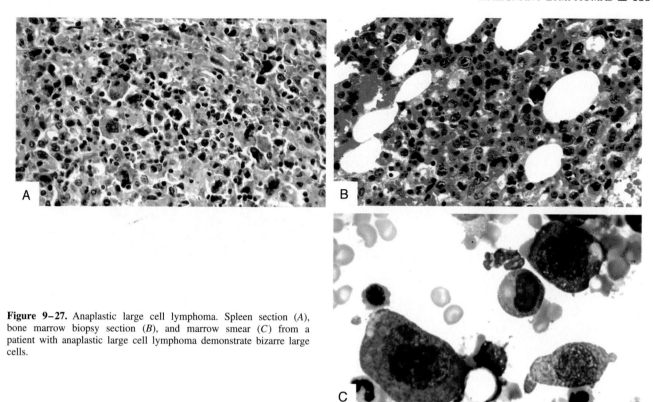

Figure 9–27. Anaplastic large cell lymphoma. Spleen section (*A*), bone marrow biopsy section (*B*), and marrow smear (*C*) from a patient with anaplastic large cell lymphoma demonstrate bizarre large cells.

Table 9–2
CLINICAL BEHAVIOR OF NON-HODGKIN'S
LYMPHOID MALIGNANCIES

Low Risk	
B Cell	*T Cell*
Small lymphocytic lymphoma/CLL	Large granular cell leukemia
Lymphoplasmacytic	Mycosis fungoides/Sézary
Hairy cell leukemia	syndrome
Marginal zone lymphomas	
Follicular lymphomas, small and mixed	
Intermediate Risk	
B Cell	*T Cell*
Prolymphocytic leukemia	Prolymphocytic leukemia
Mantle cell lymphoma	Peripheral T-cell lymphoma
Follicular lymphoma, large cell	Angioimmunoblastic lymphoma
Large cell lymphoma, diffuse	NK-like lymphoma
Plasma cell myeloma	Anaplastic large cell lymphoma
High Risk	
B Cell	*T Cell*
Precursor B-lymphoblastic leukemia/lymphoma	Precursor T-lymphoblast leukemia/lymphoma
Burkitt's and Burkitt's-like lymphoma/B-cell leukemia	Adult T-cell leukemia/lymphoma
Plasma cell leukemia	

CLL = chronic lymphoid leukemia; NK = natural killer.

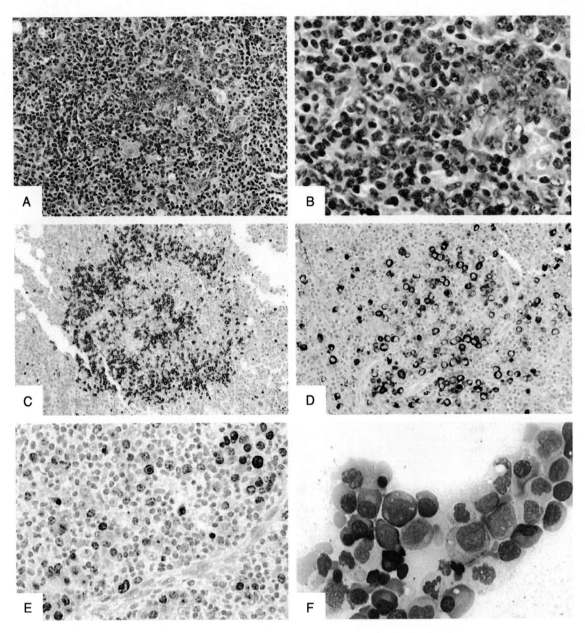

Figure 9–28. A human herpes virus 8 (HHV-8) associated plasmablastic lymphoma in a patient with AIDS. Bone marrow biopsy sections demonstrate an aggregate of immature cells (*A* and *B*) expressing CD20 (*C*), Ig kappa light chain (*D*), and HHV-8 (*E*). Bone marrow smear (*F*) shows increased number of mature and immature plasma cells.

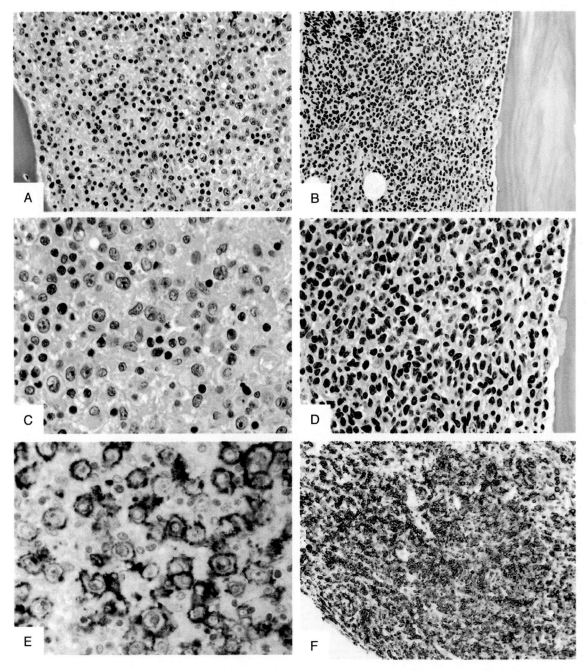

Figure 9–29. The left column (*A*, *C*, and *E*) represents bone marrow sections from a patient with large cell lymphoma. The tumor cells express CD20 (*E*). The right column (*B*, *D*, and *F*) represents bone marrow biopsy sections from the same patient following chemotherapy. There is an atypical paratrabecular lymphoid aggregate consisting of small lymphocytes, expressing CD3 (*F*). No large CD20-positive cells were found, indicating remission with a reactive T-cell process.

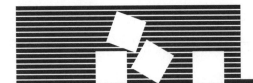

CHAPTER 10

Monoclonal Gammopathy

Monoclonal gammopathy or plasma cell dyscrasia define conditions that are the result of monoclonal proliferation of plasma cells and/or of Ig-secreting B lymphocytes. The major subtypes of plasma cell dyscrasia consist of:

1. Monoclonal gammopathy of undetermined significance ("benign" monoclonal gammopathy)
2. Plasmacytoma
3. Plasma cell myeloma (multiple myeloma) and plasma cell leukemia
4. Waldenström's macroglobulinemia and heavy chain disorders
5. Light chain–associated amyloidosis

MONOCLONAL GAMMOPATHY OF UNDETERMINED SIGNIFICANCE

Monoclonal gammopathy of undetermined significance (MGUS) is an indolent condition characterized by less than 3 g/dL monoclonal Ig in the serum, lack or trace amounts of Bence Jones protein in the urine, 5% or less plasma cells in the bone marrow (Figure 10–1), and lack of osteolytic lesions, hypercalcemia, renal failure, and anemia.

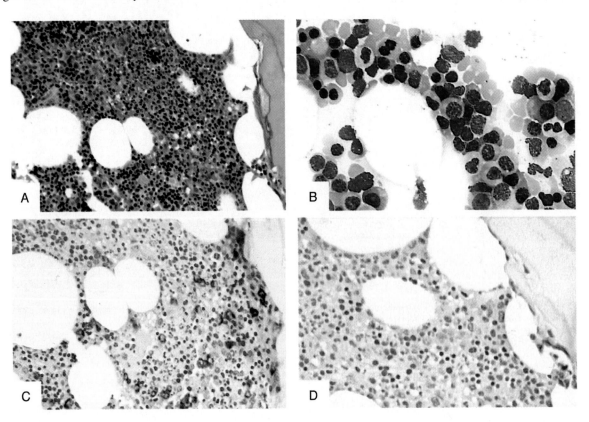

Figure 10–1. Monoclonal gammopathy of undetermined significance (MGUS). Bone marrow biopsy section (*A*) and marrow smear (*B*) demonstrate scattered plasma cells. Immunoperoxidase stains on the biopsy sections show numerous lambda light chain–positive plasma cells (*C*), whereas kappa light chain–positive plasma cells are extremely rare (*D*).

PLASMACYTOMA

Plasmacytoma is a solitary monoclonal plasmacytic proliferation affecting soft tissue or bone. The oral cavity and upper respiratory tract are the prominent sites. Plasmacytomas consist of sheets of monomorphic population of mature or immature plasma cells expressing one type (kappa or lambda) of Ig light chain (Figure 10–2). A significant proportion of patients with plasmacytoma (ranging from 15% to 55% in various reports) will eventually develop plasma cell myeloma.

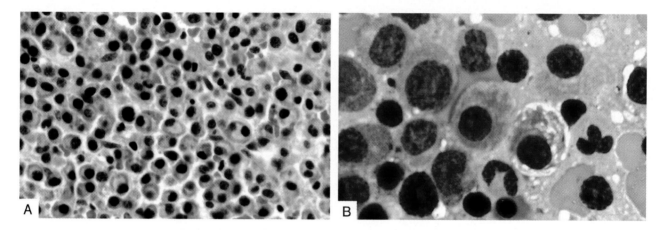

Figure 10–2. Plasmacytoma. Bone biopsy section (*A*) and aspirate (*B*) from a patient with solitary bone lesion demonstrate sheets of plasma cells, some of which show cytoplasmic vacuoles.

PLASMA CELL MYELOMA

Plasma cell myeloma, or multiple myeloma (MM), or myelomatosis is a monoclonal plasma cell disorder that affects bone marrow in multiple foci (Figure 10–3). There is an overproduction of monoclonal Ig or Ig light chain often associated with multiple osteolytic lesions, hypercalcemia, abnormal renal function, anemia, and increased susceptibility to infection. Blood smears often show red blood cell rouleaux formation. The osteosclerotic type of MM has been associated with POEMS syndrome. POEMS stands for polyneuropathy, organomegaly, endocrinopathy, monoclonal protein, and skin alterations.

Bone marrow shows an increased number of plasma cells. Plasma cells often appear in clusters, but sometimes display a diffuse or interstitial infiltration (Figures 10–4 and 10–5; see Figure 10–3). They demonstrate a wide spectrum of morphology ranging from blast-like plasma cells (plasma blasts) to large, immature, atypical forms or mature normal-appearing plasma cells (Figures 10–6 to 10–8). Binucleated or multinucleated forms may be present. Dutcher bodies (nuclear inclusions) are sometimes present but are not pathognomic features of a monoclonal process (Figure 10–9). Plasma cells in some cases may show a few or several prominent cytoplasmic vacuoles or may contain Ig crystals (Figures 10–10 and 10–11). Approximately 10% of the MM patients may show focal or extensive bone marrow fibrosis.

The criteria established by the National Cancer Institute (NCI) and the Eastern Cooperative Oncology Group (ECOG) require the presence of monoclonal serum and/or urine protein and evidence of plasmacytoma or marrow plasmacytosis of above 5% (NCI) to above 10% (ECOG). Plasma cells express CD38, CD138, and cytoplasmic monoclonal Ig, but may also demonstrate positive reaction for antigens that are typically associated with myelomonocytic cells, B cells, or T cells, such as CD13, CD14, CD10, CD2 and CD3, and CD56.

The most common chromosomal abnormalities are monosomy 13 and 16; trisomy 3, 5, 9, and 15; and t(8; 14) translocation.

Text continued on page 144

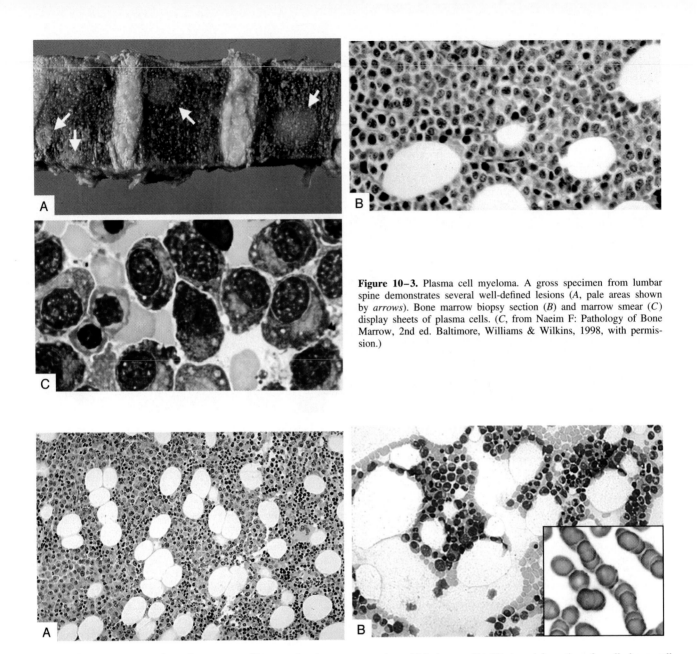

Figure 10–3. Plasma cell myeloma. A gross specimen from lumbar spine demonstrates several well-defined lesions (*A*, pale areas shown by *arrows*). Bone marrow biopsy section (*B*) and marrow smear (*C*) display sheets of plasma cells. (*C*, from Naeim F: Pathology of Bone Marrow, 2nd ed. Baltimore, Williams & Wilkins, 1998, with permission.)

Figure 10–4. Plasma cell myeloma. Bone marrow biopsy section demonstrates an interstitial plasma cell infiltrate and formation of small plasma cell clusters (*A*). Bone marrow smear shows plasma cells mixed with normal hematopoietic precursors (*B*). The inset shows a blood smear with RBC rouleaux formation.

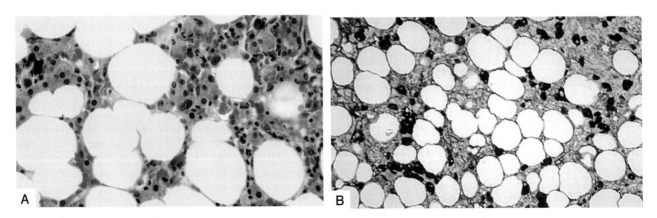

Figure 10–5. Plasma cell myeloma. *A*, Bone marrow biopsy section demonstrates an interstitial plasma cell infiltrate and formation of small plasma cell clusters. *B*, Immunoperoxidase stain shows numerous kappa light chain–positive plasma cells. Only rare cells expressed lambda light chain (results not shown).

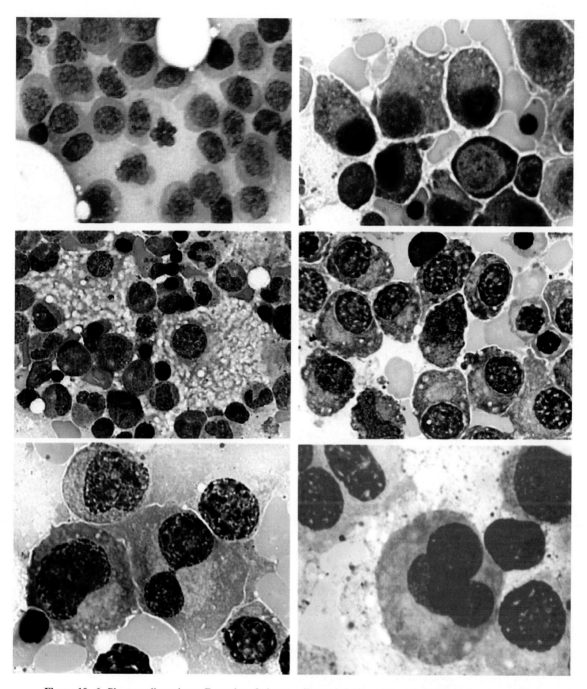

Figure 10–6. Plasma cell myeloma. Examples of plasma cell morphologic variations in monoclonal gammopathies.

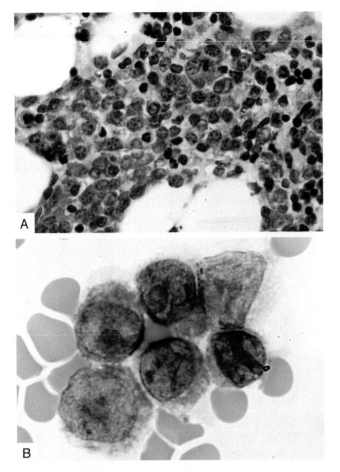

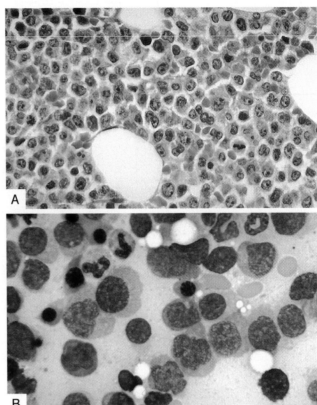

Figure 10–8. Plasma cell myeloma. Bone marrow biopsy section (*A*) and marrow smear (*B*) demonstrate sheets of atypical plasma cells with nuclear folding or convolution.

Figure 10–7. Plasma cell myeloma. Bone marrow biopsy section (*A*) and marrow smear (*B*) demonstrate clusters of immature blast-like plasma cells (plasma blasts).

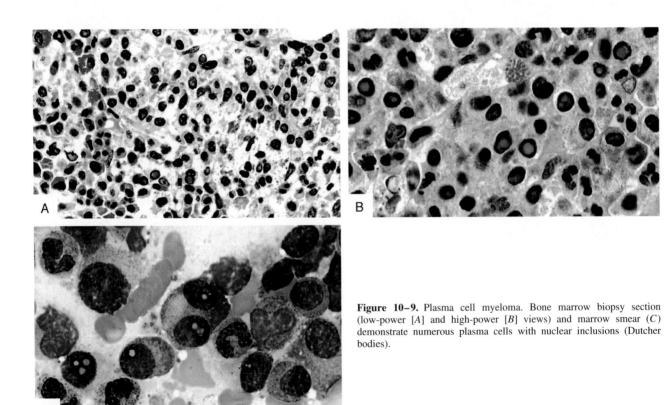

Figure 10–9. Plasma cell myeloma. Bone marrow biopsy section (low-power [*A*] and high-power [*B*] views) and marrow smear (*C*) demonstrate numerous plasma cells with nuclear inclusions (Dutcher bodies).

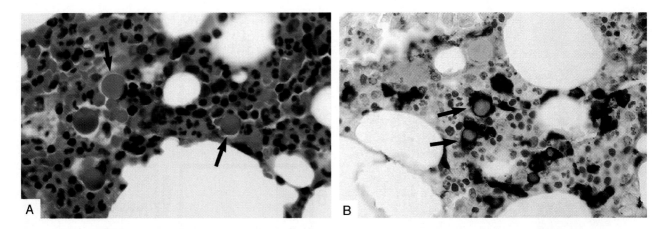

Figure 10–10. Plasma cell myeloma. *A*, Bone marrow biopsy section demonstrates numerous cells with round eosinophilic cytoplasmic inclusions (Russell bodies, *arrows*). *B*, Immunoperoxidase stain shows Ig kappa expression by these cells (*arrows*). Several small Ig kappa–positive plasma cells are also present.

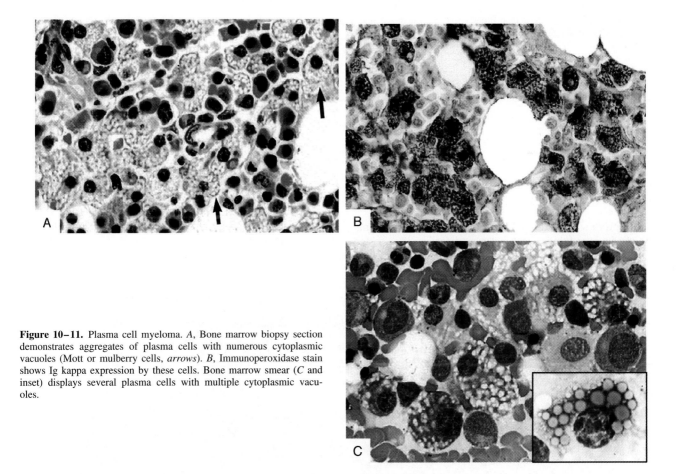

Figure 10–11. Plasma cell myeloma. *A*, Bone marrow biopsy section demonstrates aggregates of plasma cells with numerous cytoplasmic vacuoles (Mott or mulberry cells, *arrows*). *B*, Immunoperoxidase stain shows Ig kappa expression by these cells. Bone marrow smear (*C* and inset) displays several plasma cells with multiple cytoplasmic vacuoles.

PLASMA CELL LEUKEMIA

Plasma cell leukemia occurs in about 3% to 4% of MM patients. The criterion proposed for the diagnosis of plasma cell leukemia is greater than 20% plasma cells in the peripheral blood differential count or an absolute plasma cell count of $2000/\mu L$ (Figure 10–12). Plasma cell leukemia is mostly of the IgD or IgE type.

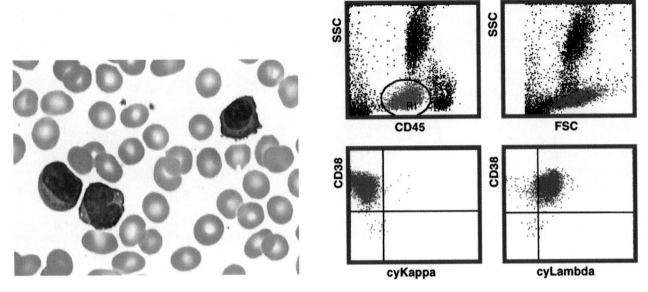

Figure 10–12. Plasma cell leukemia. Blood smear *(left)* demonstrates atypical plasma cells. Flow cytometry *(right)* shows a population of CD38/Igλ expressing cells, consistent with a monoclonal plasma cell population.

WALDENSTRÖM'S MACROGLOBULINEMIA

Waldenström's macroglobulinema (WM) is a monoclonal IgM-producing lymphoproliferative disorder manifested by lymphadenopathy, hepatomegaly, splenomegaly, and bone marrow involvement. This disorder in most instances consists of lymphoplasmacytic cells (lymphoplasmacytic lymphoma), but may also be associated with other lymphoid malignancies (Figures 10–13 to 10–15) (see Chapter 9).

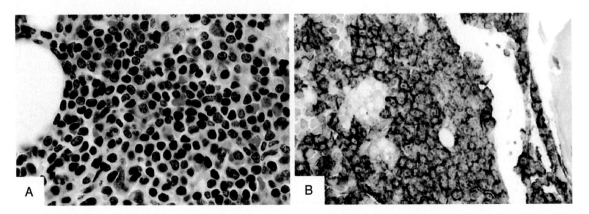

Figure 10–13. Waldenström's macroglobulinemia. Bone marrow biopsy section demonstrates a lymphoplasmacytic infiltrate *(A)*. Immunoperoxidase stains show the expression of IgM *(B)* and kappa light chain *(C)* by the majority of the infiltrating cells. Plasma cells and scattered lymphoplasmacytic cells are also positive for CD138 *(D)*.

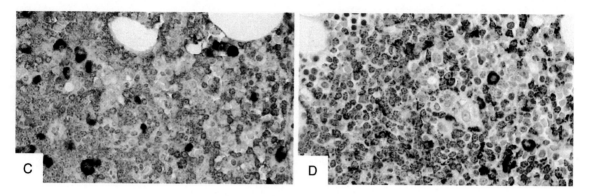

Figure 10–13. *Continued*

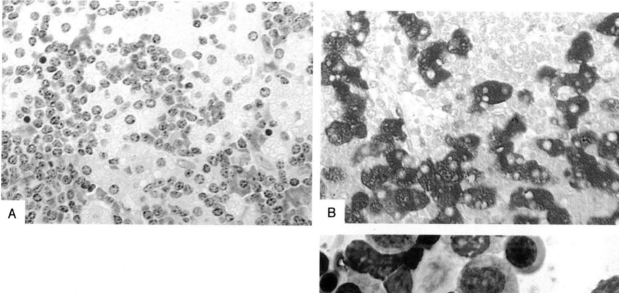

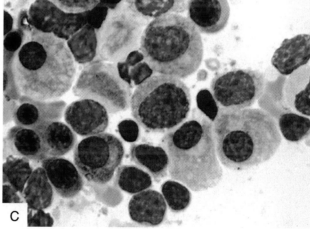

Figure 10–14. Waldenström's macroglobulinemia. Bone marrow biopsy section demonstrates a lymphoplasmacytic infiltrate with aggregates of plasma cells with abundant pale vacuolated cytoplasm (*A*). The plasma cells express Ig kappa light chain by immunoperoxidase stain (*B*). Bone marrow smear displays a lymphoplasmacytic infiltrate with vacuolated plasma cells (*C*).

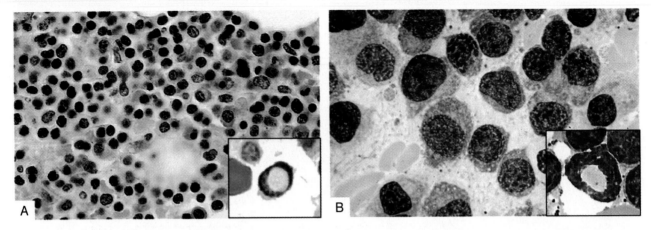

Figure 10–15. Waldenström's macroglobulinemia. Bone marrow biopsy section (*A*) and marrow smear (*B*) demonstrate a lymphoplasmacytic infiltrate. Insets show plasma cells with nuclear inclusion (Dutcher bodies).

LIGHT CHAIN–ASSOCIATED AMYLOIDOSIS

Immunoglobulin light chain (primary) amyloidosis is a systemic disorder associated with plasma cell dyscrasia. Ig lambda light chain is involved more frequently than the kappa light chain (Figure 10–16). Approximately 60% of the cases may also show a low level of monoclonal serum protein.

Bone marrow sections depict an extracellular eosinophilic amyloid deposit, which is positive by Congo red stain and appears as a birefringent apple-green color under a polarized light (Figure 10–16). The amyloid deposits are found predominantly within and around the vessel walls. In some cases, bone marrow shows a monoclonal plasmacytosis detected by the immunoenzyme stains (see Figure 10–16).

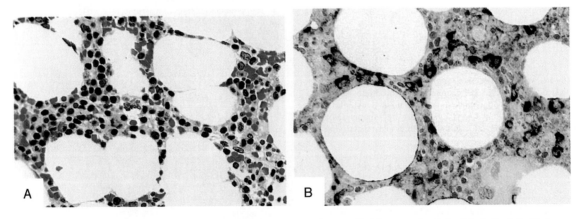

Figure 10–16. Amyloidosis. Bone marrow biopsy section demonstrates scattered plasma cells (*A*) expressing Ig lambda light chain (*B*, immunoperoxidase stain). One of the sclerotic blood vessels in the biopsy section (*C*) displays an apple-green birefringent deposit by Congo red stain (*D*).

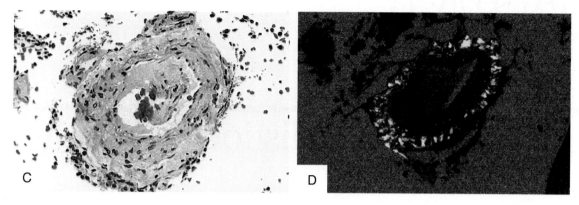

Figure 10–16. *Continued*

CLINICAL ASPECTS

The average age of patients with plasma cell disorders is around 55 and the incidence increases with age. Approximately 10% of the patients with MGUS develop plasma cell myeloma at 5 years, and the rate almost doubles at 10 years.

Several prognostic factors have been identified in patients with MM, and a number of staging systems have been developed for the identification of patients with poor prognosis. In general, high plasma cell mass, severe anemia, renal failure, elevated levels of serum β_2-microglobulin, immunoglobulin and calcium, and systemic amyloidosis are associated with poor prognosis. Also, patients with plasma cell leukemia have an aggressive clinical course and poor response to chemotherapy.

DIFFERENTIAL DIAGNOSIS

Differential diagnosis includes reactive plasmacytosis, immunoblastic lymphoma, and metastatic carcinoma. Reactive plasmacytosis in excess of 10% may occur in a number of conditions, such as autoimmune disorders, immunodeficiency syndromes, immune reaction to drugs, Castleman's disease, myelodysplastic syndromes, Hodgkin's lymphoma, viral infections, and postchemotherapy. In these conditions, plasma cells are generally mature and polyclonal. Neoplastic cells in immunoblastic lymphoma usually express B cell–associated markers, such as CD19 and CD20, whereas plasma cells lack expression of these molecules. Metastatic carcinoma cells are cytokeratin-positive and Ig-negative.

Selected References

Alexanian R, Weber D, Liu F: Differential diagnosis of monoclonal gammopathies. Arch Pathol Lab Med 123:108, 1999.

Baldini L, Guffanti A, Cesana BM, et al: Role of different hematologic variables in defining the risk of malignant transformation in monoclonal gammopathy. Blood 87:912, 1996.

Bartl R, Frisch, B: Clinical significance of bone marrow biopsy and plasma cell morphology in MM and MGUS. Pathol Biol 47:158, 1999.

Bergsagel PL, Smith AM, Szczepek A, et al: In multiple myeloma, clonotypic B lymphocytes are detectable among CD19+ peripheral blood cells expressing CD38, CD56, and monotypic Ig light chain. Blood 85:436, 1995.

Blade J, Kyle RA, Greipp R: Presenting features and prognosis in 72 patients with multiple myeloma who were younger than 40 years. Br J Haematol 93:345, 1996.

Feiner HD, Bannan M, Marsh E, et al: Monoclonal gammopathy of undetermined significance: A morphologic and immunophenotypic study of the bone marrow. Modern Pathol 5:372, 1992.

Greipp PR: Advances in the diagnosis and management of myeloma. Semin Hematol 29(Suppl 2):24, 1992.

Kyle RA: Why better prognostic factors for multiple myeloma are needed. Blood 83:1713, 1994.

Kyle RA, Gertz MA, Greipp PR, et al: Long-term survival (10 years or more) in 30 patients with primary amyloidosis. Blood 93:1062, 1999.

Naeim F: Pathology of Bone Marrow. Baltimore, Williams & Wilkins, 1997, p 328.

Saeed SM, Stock-Novack D, Pohlod R, et al: Prognostic correlation of plasma cell acid phosphatase and β-glucuronidase in multiple myeloma: A Southwest Oncology Group study. Blood 78:3281, 1991.

Wu SS-H, Brady K, Anderson JJ, et al: The predictive value of bone marrow morphologic characteristics and immunostaining in primary (AL) amyloidosis. Am J Clin Pathol 96:95, 1991.

CHAPTER 11

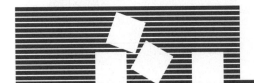

Histiocytic Disorders

Histiocytes are derived from committed stem cells (colony forming units–monocyte, CFU-M) in the bone marrow by passing through maturation stages of monoblast, promonocyte, and monocyte. They appear in many different morphologic forms and functional capacities (see Figure 11–1). The majority of currently known monocytic/histiocytic disorders are quantitative. They often lead to increased numbers of monocytic/histiocytic cells in the bone marrow and/or peripheral blood (Table 11–1). In this chapter, the focus is on the proliferative histiocytic syndromes and lysosomal storage diseases.

Table 11–1

DISORDERS ASSOCIATED WITH
MONOCYTOSIS/HISTIOCYTOSIS

Langerhans cell histiocytosis
Hemophagocytic histiocytosis
    Familial
    Infection-associated
    Cancer-associated
    Others (i.e., Chédiak-Higashi syndrome)
Sinus histiocytosis with massive lymphadenopathy
Granulomatous disorders
Malignant monocytic/histiocytic disorders
Lysosomal storage diseases

HISTIOCYTOSIS

The proliferative histiocytic syndromes are divided into three major classes: Langerhans cell histiocytosis (class I histiocytosis); reactive histiocytic/macrophage proliferations (class II histiocytosis); and malignant monocytic/histiocytic disorders (class III histiocytosis).

Langerhans Cell Histiocytosis

Langerhans cell histiocytosis (LCH), also known as *histiocytosis X*, embraces a wide variety of clinicopathologic conditions, such as *eosinophilic granuloma, Letterer-Siwe disease, Hand-Schüller-Christian disease*, and *Hashimoto-Pritzker syndrome*. Langerhans cells are a subclass of dendritic cells, which are derived from bone marrow stem cells committed to produce monocytic/histiocytic precursors.

Bone marrow sections demonstrate focal or diffuse infiltration of large mononuclear cells with abundant, finely granular or vacuolated eosinophilic cytoplasm, and an oval, irregular, folded or indented nucleus (Figures 11–1 to 11–5). Nucleoli are inconspicuous and mitotic figures are absent or extremely rare. Hemophagocytosis is usually infrequent or absent. The infiltrate is often mixed with inflammatory cells, particularly eosinophils (see Figures 11–4 and 11–5). Multinucleated giant cells are sometimes present (see Figure 11–5). Chronic lesions show more fibrosis and may appear less cellular. Marrow smears show increased numbers of large mononuclear cells with abundant cytoplasm, and round or irregular nucleus (see Figures 11–1, 11–2, and 11–4). The cytoplasm is sometimes vacuolated and may depict elongated projections.

The Langerhans cells express CD1 and S100, are positive for ATPase, alpha-D-mannosidase, and bind to peanut lectin (see Figures 11–2 and 11–3). Electron microscopy demonstrates characteristic tennis racket–shaped cytoplasmic *Birbeck* granules (Figure 11–6).

Clinical Aspects

Patients with LCH are predominantly young. Over 90% of the patients are diagnosed before age 30 and over 70% are younger than 10. The most frequent sites of involvement are skin, bone (and bone marrow), lymph nodes, spleen, and liver. Poor prognostic factors include age younger than 2 years, multiple organ involvement, and pancytopenia.

Differential Diagnosis

Differential diagnosis of LCH includes reactive histiocytosis, granulomas, Hodgkin's disease, large cell lymphoma, clear cell carcinoma, and mast cell disease. In questionable cases the presence of Birbeck granules and the expression of CD1 and S100 help to confirm the diagnosis.

Hemophagocytic Syndromes

Hemophagocytic syndromes are a group of histiocytic disorders characterized by the proliferation of reactive non-Langerhans cell histiocytes with hemophagocytic activities (Figure 11–7). These include familial (primary) hemophagocytic lymphohistiocytosis, infection- and cancer-associated hemophagocytic syndromes, and sinus histiocytosis with massive lymphadenopathy.

Familial Hemophagocytic Lymphohistiocytosis

Familial (primary) hemophagocytic lymphohistiocytosis is an autosomal recessive disorder characterized by fever, hepatosplenomegaly, cytopenia of at least two lineages, hypertriglyceridemia and/or hypofibrinogenemia, and bone marrow hemophagocytosis, without evidence of infection or malignancy. The incidence is sporadic, and at onset, family history is often negative.

Bone marrow samples reveal variable numbers of histiocytes, some of which show evidence of hemophagocytosis, particularly erythrophagocytosis (Figure 11–8). Histiocytes are mature and bland-appearing with no cytologic atypia. These cells, unlike the Langerhans cells, are strongly positive for nonspecific esterase, lysozyme, and CD68, are negative for CD1 and S100, and do not demonstrate Birbeck granules. There is also evidence of bone marrow lymphocytosis with high proportion of T lymphocytes. The extent of bone marrow involvement varies; in the early stages, bone marrow examination may show minimal nondiagnostic changes, whereas in the advanced stages there are numerous phagocytic histiocytes and often a reduction in the bone marrow cellularity.

Infection-Associated Hemophagocytic Syndrome

A wide variety of microorganisms, such as viruses, bacteria, fungi, and rickettsias, are able to induce reactive histiocytosis with hemophagocytic activities (Figure 11–9). The reactive histiocytes are most commonly found in the bone marrow, but they may also be present in the spleen, liver, and lymph nodes. Variable proportions of the histiocytes contain phagocytosed erythrocytes and/or other hematopoietic cells. Bone marrow cellularity is often reduced in advanced cases.

Cancer-Associated Hemophagocytosis

Hemophagocytosis has been reported in association with a wide variety of malignancies, particulaly T-cell lymphomas/leukemias (Figure 11–10). The combination of hemophagocytosis and the presence of tumor cells may simulate malignant histiocytosis. However, the phagocytic cells are usually reactive histiocytes containing erythrocytes and/or other hematopoietic cells, though some of the neoplastic cells may also show hemophagocytosis.

Clinical Aspects

The reactive hemophagocytic disorders are characterized by cytopenia (anemia or pancytopenia), hyperlipidemia, elevated serum triglycerides, and hepatosplenomegaly. Lymphadenopathy may also be present. The clinical course may be complicated by coagulation abnormalities, hepatic dysfunction, and, sometimes, renal failure.

The clinicopathologic similarities between hemophagocytic syndromes and accelerated phase of Chédiak-Higashi syndrome (see Chapter 12), and their association with immunodeficiency states, suggest a common pathway of an abnormal immune response leading to the proliferation and activation of the histiocytes.

Differential Diagnosis

Primary hemophagocytic lymphohistiocytosis is distinguished from the infection- and cancer-associated variants by the presence of family history and the absence of infection or malignancy. The reactive hemophagocytic syndromes do not show the cytologic atypism that is usually observed in histiocytic malignancies. Some of the advanced cases of Chédiak-Higashi syndrome may demonstrate hemophagocytic histiocytosis.

Sinus Histiocytosis With Massive Lymphadenopathy

Sinus histiocytosis with massive lymphadenopathy (Rosai-Dorfman syndrome) is a benign chronic sinus histiocytosis of the cervical lymph nodes characterized by the presence of marked emperipolesis (engulfed lymphocytes within the cytoplasm of histiocytes).

Granulomas

Granulomas are collections of epithelioid histiocytes often surrounded by lymphocytes and plasma cells (Figure 11–11). The most frequent causes of granuloma are sarcoidosis, and mycobacterial and fungal infections. However, other infectious and noninfectious conditions may develop bone marrow granuloma (see Chapter 2).

Monocytic/Histiocytic Malignancies

Monocytic premalignant and malignant conditions are discussed in Chapters 3 to 5. Histiocytic malignancies are rare and may appear as solid tumors (histiocytic lymphoma) or diffusely involve the reticuloendothelial system (malignant histiocytosis, AML-M5c) (Figure 11–12). Malignant tumors of the dendritic cells are extremely rare.

Text continued on page 155

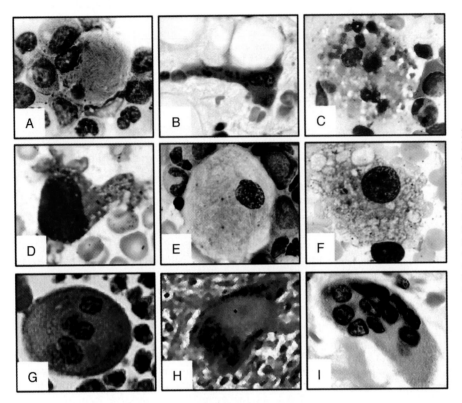

Figure 11–1. Macrophage/histiocytic cells. Bone marrow smears demonstrate a variety of macrophage/histiocytic cells. A sea-blue histiocyte (*A*), an iron-loaded histiocyte (*B*), a macrophage containing cell debris and iron particles (*C*), a Langerhans dendritic cell with elongated cytoplasmic projections (*D*), a Gaucher cell (*E*), a vacuolated macrophage from a patient with Niemann-Pick disease (*F*), a multinucleated histiocyte in a patient with Langerhans cell histiocytosis (*G*), a multinucleated giant form in a patient with tuberculosis, and an osteoclast (*I*) are demonstrated in this figure.

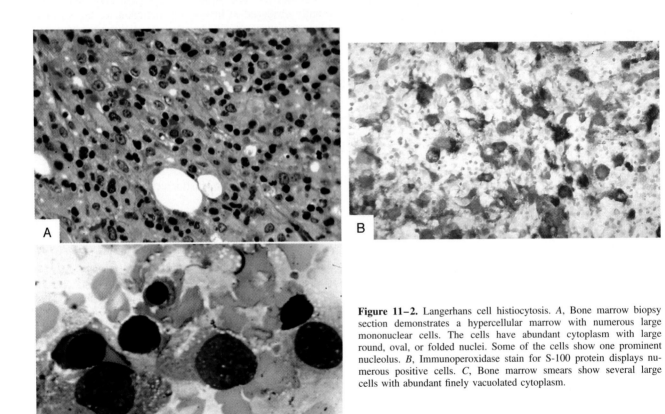

Figure 11–2. Langerhans cell histiocytosis. *A,* Bone marrow biopsy section demonstrates a hypercellular marrow with numerous large mononuclear cells. The cells have abundant cytoplasm with large round, oval, or folded nuclei. Some of the cells show one prominent nucleolus. *B,* Immunoperoxidase stain for S-100 protein displays numerous positive cells. *C,* Bone marrow smears show several large cells with abundant finely vacuolated cytoplasm.

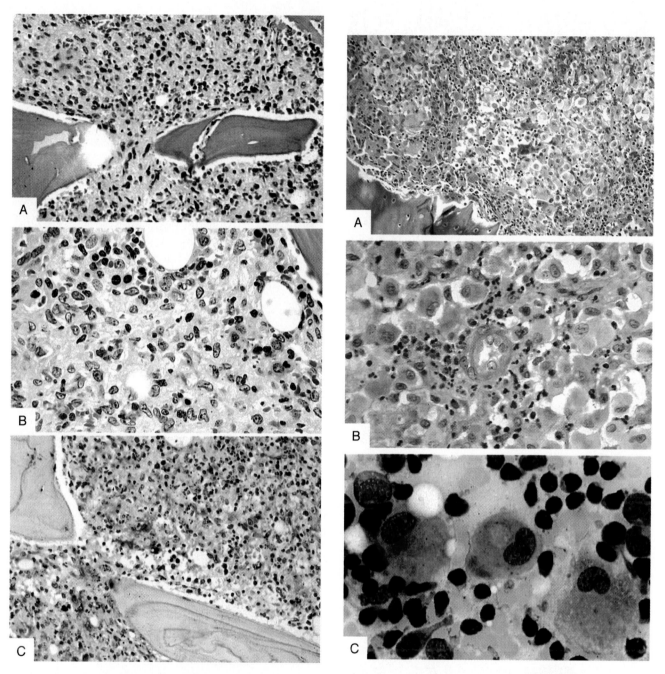

Figure 11–3. Langerhans cell histiocytosis. Bone marrow biopsy section demonstrates a hypercellular marrow with numerous large mononuclear cells (low-power [A] and high-power [B] views). The cells have abundant cytoplasm with large round, oval, or folded nuclei. C, Immunoperoxidase stain for CD1c shows numerous positive cells.

Figure 11–4. Langerhans cell histiocytosis. Bone marrow biopsy section (A and B) and marrow smear (C) demonstrate large mononuclear cells with abundant cytoplasm and large round, oval, or folded nuclei. Numerous eosinophils are also present (A and B).

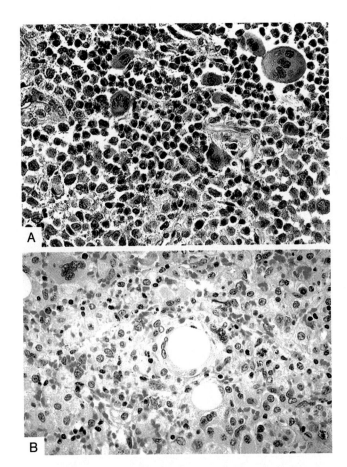

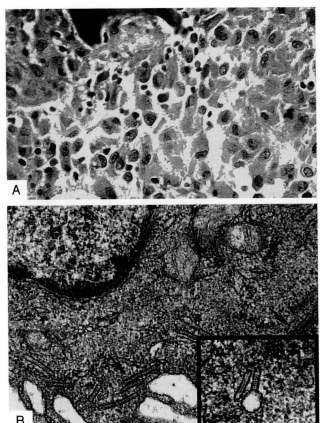

Figure 11–5. Langerhans cell histiocytosis. Bone marrow biopsy sections demonstrate sheets of histiocytes with multinucleated forms and increased eosinophils (*A*), or only aggregates of histiocytes (*B*).

Figure 11–6. Langerhans cell histiocytosis. *A*, Bone marrow biopsy section demonstrates sheets of Langerhans cells. *B*, Electron micrograph of a Langerhans cell shows Birbeck granules. The inset displays a tennis racket–like structure. (*B*, Courtesy of Sunita Bhuta, M.D., Department of Pathology and Laboratory Medicine, UCLA Medical Center.)

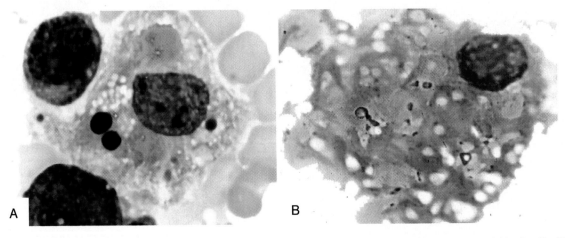

Figure 11–7. Hemophagocytic macrophages. Bone marrow samples demonstrate macrophages with phagocytosed red blood cells (RBCs) and nucleated cells (marrow smears [*A–C*] and biopsy section [*D*]). A sea-blue histiocyte is shown in *B*, and *D* is an iron stain displaying several iron-loaded macrophages with phagocytosed RBCs. (*A–C*, from Naeim F: Pathology of Bone Marrow, 2nd ed. Baltimore, Williams & Wilkins, 1998, with permission.)

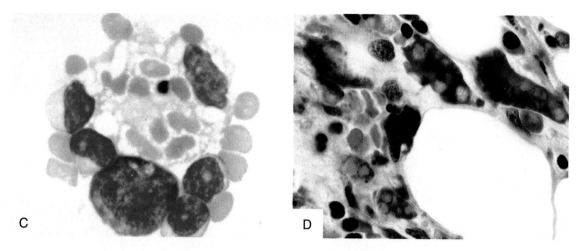

Figure 11–7. *Continued*

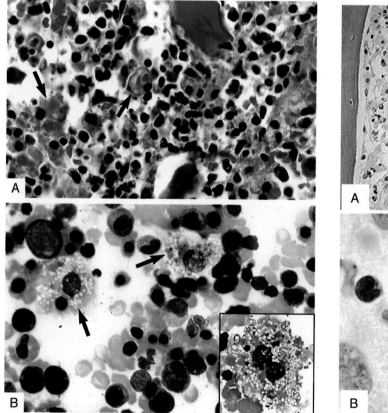

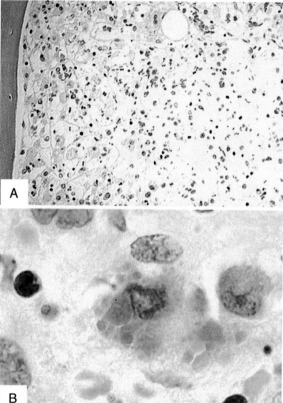

Figure 11–8. Familial hemophagocytic lymphohistiocytosis (FHLH). *A,* Bone marrow biopsy section from a 3-year-old boy with FHLH demonstrates several macrophages with phagocytosed erythrocytes (*arrows*). Macrophages with phagocytosed RBCs and cellular debris are displayed in the bone marrow smears (*B, arrows,* and inset).

Figure 11–9. Infection-associated hemophagocytosis. Bone marrow biopsy section from a patient with Epstein-Barr virus (EBV) infection demonstrates increased numbers of histiocytes (*A*) with macrophages containing large numbers of erythrocytes (*B*). (From Naeim F: Pathology of Bone Marrow, 2nd ed. Baltimore, Williams & Wilkins, 1998, with permission.)

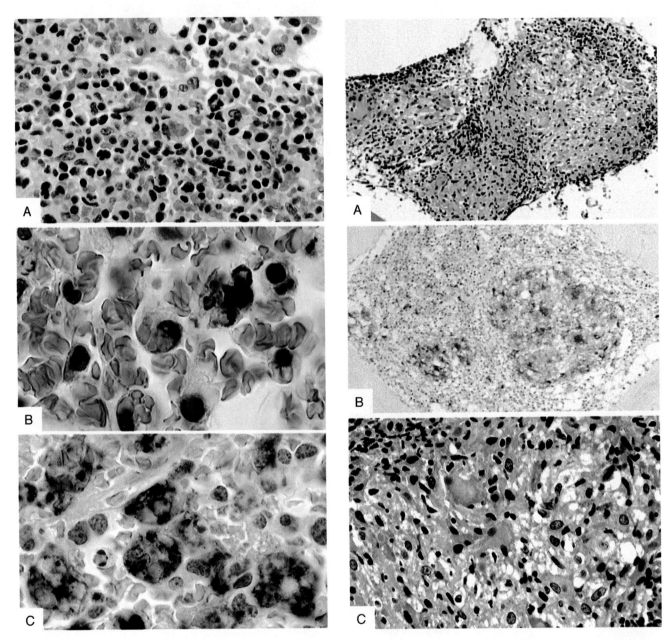

Figure 11–10. Cancer-associated hemophagocytosis. Bone marrow biopsy section from a patient with a history of T-cell lymphoma demonstrates lymphomatous involvement (*A*). A high-power view displays several RBC-containing macrophages (*B*). The macrophages are stained for CD68 by the immunoperoxidase technique (*C*).

Figure 11–11. Granulomas. Bone marrow biopsy section from a patient with sarcoidosis demonstrates several small granulomas consisting of epithelioid histiocytes surrounded by chronic inflammatory cells. Low-power view (*A*), immunoperoxidase stain for CD68 (*B*), and high-power view (*C*).

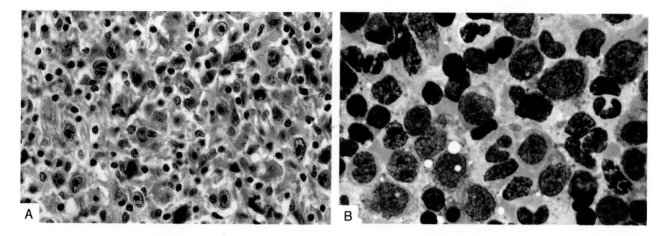

Figure 11–12. Histiocytic malignancy. Bone marrow biopsy section (*A*) and marrow smear (*B*) from a patient with a history of histiocytic lymphoma demonstrate bone marrow involvement. The neoplastic cells are large and show a variable amount of cytoplasm and large, convoluted nuclei. They were strongly positive for CD68 and lysozyme and negative for the lymphoid markers (results not shown).

LYSOSOMAL STORAGE DISEASES

Hereditary deficiencies of the lysosomal enzymes result in accumulation of the glycolipid or glycoprotein substrates in macrophages and the development of lysosomal storage diseases. Various subclasses of lysosomal storage diseases have been described. In this chapter, Gaucher's and Niemann-Pick diseases are discussed because of their association with significant bone marrow pathology.

Gaucher's Disease

Gaucher's disease is an autosomal recessive condition caused by the deficiency of glucocerebrosidase and accumulation of glucocerebroside in tissue macrophages (Gaucher cells) in the reticuloendothelial system, including liver, spleen, bone marrow, and lymph nodes. The glucocerebrosidase gene complex is located at region q21 of chromosome 1.

Gaucher cells are characterized by abundant cytoplasm with wrinkles or striations due to accumulation of glucocerebroside molecules (Figures 11–13 and 11–14). The cytoplasm is periodic acid-Schiff (PAS)-positive and depicts strong tartrate-resistant acid phosphatase (TRAP) activity. The nucleus is small and is often pushed to one side.

Clusters or sheets of Gaucher cells are often present in bone marrow preparations (see Figure 11–14). Accumulation of Gaucher cells may be associated with bone marrow fibrosis, leading to an unsuccessful marrow aspiration.

Blood examination reveals a marked decline in leukocyte glucocerebrosidase levels, and a markedly elevated serum acid phosphatase. Mild to moderate cytopenia, particularly anemia, is often present.

Clinical Aspects

Gaucher's disease is the most prevalent lysosomal storage disease and is divided into three major clinical subtypes based on the extent of neurologic abnormalities: *nonneuropathic* (chronic adult type), *subacute neuropathic*, and *acute neuropathic*. The nonneuropathic type is the most common form and is more frequent in the Ashkenazi Jews. All three subtypes demonstrate involvement of the reticuloendothelial system.

Differential Diagnosis

Lipid-laden Gaucher-like cells may be present in other conditions, such as myelodysplastic syndromes, chronic myelogenous leukemia (CML), and other myeloproliferative disorders. Definitive diagnosis of Gaucher's disease is established by enzyme assays and molecular studies.

Niemann-Pick Disease

Niemann-Pick disease is a rare autosomal recessive disorder caused by the deficiency of sphingomyelinase. The characteristic pathologic feature of the disease is the presence of foamy macrophages (Niemann-Pick cells) in various tisues, including bone marrow (Figures 11–15 to 11–17). The Niemann-Pick cells contain lipid and lipopigment and stain intensively with iron hematoxylin. The unstained air-dried marrow smears are birefringent under polarized light.

Blood examination reveals the lack of leukocyte sphingomyelinase activity. Mild to moderate cytopenia is often present. Lymphocytes may demonstrate cytoplasmic vacuoles as a result of the accumulation of sphingomyelin.

Clinical Aspects

The decline of sphingomyelinase in Niemann-Pick disease is either primary (group I) or secondary (group II). Group I Niemann-Pick disease is divided into *neuropathic* (infantile) and *visceral* subtypes. Group II Niemann-Pick disease is less frequent and overall has a less aggressive clinical course than group I.

Differential Diagnosis

Foamy histiocytes are seen in a variety of conditions, such as Langerhans cell histiocytosis, hypercholesterolemia, Wolman's disease, and familial high-density lipoprotein deficiency. Demonstration of sphingomyelinase deficiency in leukocytes and identification of the stored sphingomyelin in foamy histiocytes establish the diagnosis of Niemann-Pick disease.

Selected References

Ben-Ezra JM, Koo CH: Langerhans' cell histiocytosis and malignancies of the M-PIRE system. Am J Clin Pathol 99:464, 1993.

Boruchoff SE, Woda BA, Pihan GA, et al: Parvovirus B19-associated hemophagocytic syndrome. Arch Intern Med 150:897, 1990.

Cline M: Histiocytes and histiocytosis. Blood 84:2840, 1994.

Dehner LP: Morphologic findings in the histiocytic syndromes. Semin Oncol 18:8, 1991.

Egeler RM, Nesbit ME: Langerhans cell histiocytosis and other disorders of monocyte-histiocyte lineage. Crit Rev Oncol Hematol 18:9, 1995.

Falini B, Pileri S, De S Olas I, et al: Peripheral T-cell lymphoma associated with hemophagocytic syndrome. Blood 75:434, 1990.

Favara BE, Feller AC, Pauli M, et al: Contemporary classification of histiocytic disorders. The WHO Committee on Histiocytic/Reticulum Cell Proliferations. Reclassification Working Group of the Histiocyte Society. Med Pediatr Oncol 29:157, 1997.

Favara BE, Jaffe R: The histopathology of Langerhans cell histiocytosis. Brit J Med 70:175, 1994.

Gogusev J, Nezelof C: Malignant histiocytosis. Histologic, cytochemical, chromosomal, and molecular data and nosologic discussion. Hematol Oncol Clin North Am 12:445, 1998.

Henter JI, Aricò M, Elinder G, et al: Familial hemophagocytic lymphohistiocytosis. Primary hemophagocytic lymphohistiocytosis. Hematol Oncol Clin North Am 12:417, 1998.

Henter J-I, Elinder G, Ost A, et al: Diagnostic guidelines for hemophagocytic lymphohistiocytosis. Sem Oncol 18:29, 1991.

Herzog KM, Tubbs RR: Langerhans cell histiocytosis. Adv Anatomic Pathol 5:347, 1998.

Incerti C: Gaucher disease; an overview. Semin Hematol 32:3, 1995.

Janka G, Imashuku S, Elinder G, et al: Infection- and malignancy-associated hemophagocytic syndromes. Secondary hemophagocytic lymphohistiocytosis. Hematol Oncol Clin North Am 12:435, 1998.

Ladisch S: Langerhans cell histiocytosis. Curr Opin Hematol 5:54, 1998.

Laurecet FM, Chapuis B, Roux-Lombard P, et al: Malignant histiocytosis in the leukemic stage: A new entity (M5c-AML) in the FAB classification? Leukemia 8:502, 1994.

Liscum L, Klansek JJ: Niemann-Pick disease type C. Curr Opin Lipidol 9:131, 1998.

Malpas JS: Langerhans cell histiocytosis in adults. Hematol Oncol Clin North Am 12:259, 1998.

Okano M, Gross TG: Epstein-Barr virus-associated hemophagocytic syndrome and fatal infectious mononucleosis. Am J Hematol 53:111, 1996.

Pastores GM: Gaucher's disease. Pathological features. Bail Clin Haematol 10:739, 1997.

Takeshita M, Kikuchi M, Ohshima K, et al: Bone marrow findings in malignant histiocytosis and/or malignant lymphoma with concurrent hemophagocytic syndrome. Leuk Lymph 12:79, 1993.

Tephan JL: Histiocytosis. Eur J Pediatr 154:600, 1995.

Velez-Yanguas MC, Warrier RP: Langerhans' cell histiocytosis. Orthoped Clin North Am 27:615, 1996.

Woda BA, Sullivan JH: Reactive histiocytic disorders. Am J Clin Pathol 99:459, 1993.

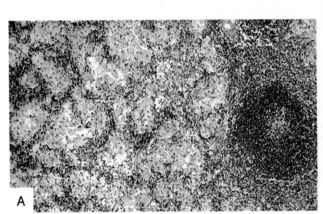
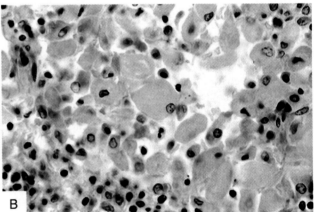

Figure 11–13. Gaucher's disease. Section of spleen demonstrates clusters of histiocytes with abundant eosinophilic cytoplasm (low-power [*A*] and high-power [*B*] views). PAS stain demonstrates accumulation of glucocerebroside molecules in membranous sheets creating cytoplasmic striations (*C*). (*A*, from Naeim F: Pathology of Bone Marrow, 2nd ed. Baltimore, Williams & Wilkins, 1998, with permission.)

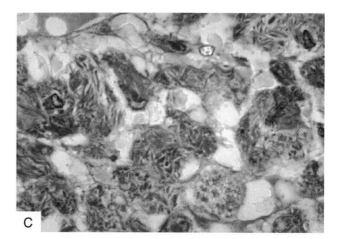

Figure 11–13. *Continued*

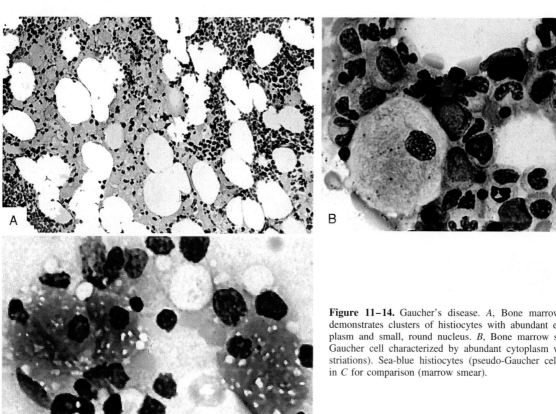

Figure 11–14. Gaucher's disease. *A,* Bone marrow biopsy section demonstrates clusters of histiocytes with abundant eosinophilic cytoplasm and small, round nucleus. *B,* Bone marrow smear shows one Gaucher cell characterized by abundant cytoplasm with wrinkles (or striations). Sea-blue histiocytes (pseudo-Gaucher cells) are presented in *C* for comparison (marrow smear).

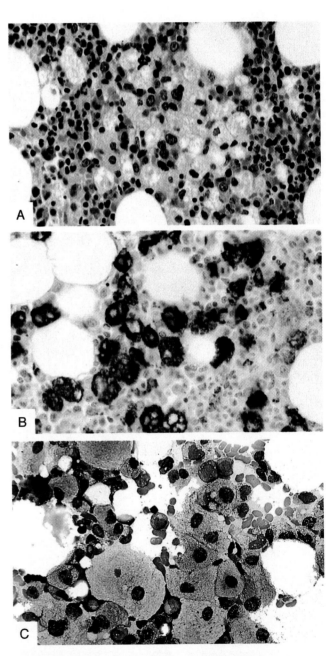

Figure 11–15. Niemann-Pick disease. Bone marrow biopsy section demonstrates replacement of the normal bone marrow cells by large, vacuolated histiocytes (low-power [*A*] and high-power [*B*] views). Bone marrow smear shows two large vacuolated histiocytes (Niemann-Pick cell [*C*]).

Figure 11–16. Niemann-Pick disease. Bone marrow biopsy section demonstrates clusters of histiocytes with abundant vacuolated cytoplasm (*A*). These cells are CD68-positive (*B*, immunoperoxidase stain). Bone marrow smear displays clusters of histiocytes with abundant, finely vacuolated cytoplasm (Niemann-Pick cells [*C*]).

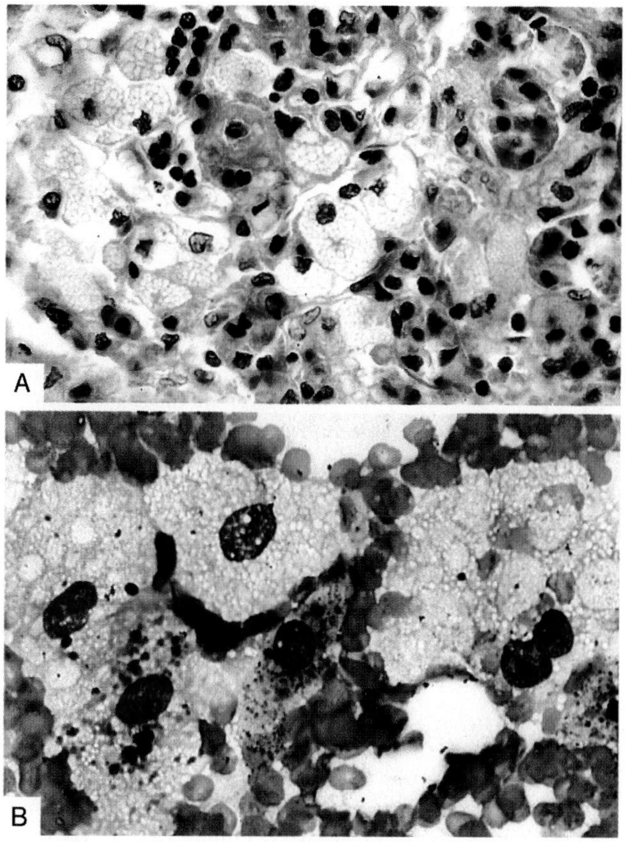

Figure 11–17. Niemann-Pick disease. Bone marrow biopsy section (*A*) and marrow smear (*B*) demonstrate several histiocytes with abundant, finely vacuolated cytoplasm (Niemann-Pick cells).

CHAPTER 12

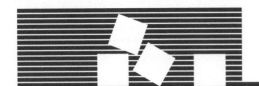

Granulocytic Disorders

ABNORMAL MORPHOLOGY

Granulocytic series may show various forms of abnormal morphology including the presence of abnormal cytoplasmic granules or inclusions, and abnormal nuclear shape or lobulation (Figure 12–1).

Cytoplasmic Granules and Inclusions

Toxic Granulation

Toxic granulation is defined as the presence of small, dark blue cytoplasmic lysosomal granules in neutrophils (see Figure 12–1). They are found in infections, burns, drug toxicity, and leukemoid reactions.

Döhle Inclusion Bodies

Döhle bodies are pear-shaped or oval aggregates of rough endoplasmic reticulum (see Figure 12–1). They appear as light blue or gray cytoplasmic inclusions with Wright's stain. Döhle bodies frequently accompany toxic granulations, but are also seen in May-Hegglin anomaly.

Alder-Reilly Anomaly

Alder-Reilly anomaly refers to the presence of dense azurophilic granules in granulocytes and, sometimes, monocytes and lymphocytes (see Figure 12–1). They are found in mucopolysaccharidoses (subtypes of lysosomal storage diseases).

Chédiak-Higashi Syndrome

This syndrome is a rare autosomal recessive disease characterized by abnormal membrane fluidity and fusion of cytoplasmic granules in leukocytes and platelets (see Figure 12–1). There are large bluish-purple cytoplasmic granules in neutrophils. Some of the advanced cases of Chédiak-Higashi syndrome may demonstrate hemophagocytic histiocytosis (see Chapter 11).

Abnormal Nuclear Morphology

Pelger-Huët Anomaly

Pelger-Huët anomaly is associated with reduced nuclear segmentation in neutrophils (see Figure 12–1). Most nuclei are band-shaped or bisegmented. Pelger-Huët anomaly is either congenital or acquired. The acquired anomaly is seen in myelodysplastic syndromes (MDS), chronic myelogenous leukemia (CML), and some cases of lymphomas.

Hypersegmented Neutrophils

Neutrophilic nuclear hypersegmentation (more than five lobes) is observed in megaloblastic anemia as well as MDS, CML, and chronic infections (see Figure 12–1). A rare autosomal dominant hereditary condition has been reported with giant hypersegmented neutrophils.

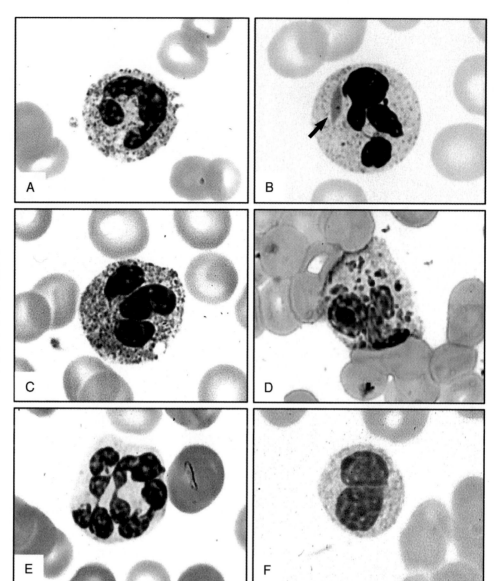

Figure 12–1. Abnormal neutrophils. Examples of abnormal cytoplasmic structures are demonstrated as toxic granulation (*A*), Döhle inclusion bodies (*B, arrow*), Alder-Reilly anomaly in mucopolysaccharidosis (*C*), and cytoplasmic inclusions in Chédiak-Higashi syndrome (*D*). Examples of abnormal nuclear morphology are shown as hypersegmentation (*E*) and hyposegmentation (*F*).

CONGENITAL NEUTROPENIA

Congenital neutropenias consist of autosomal-recessive (Kostmann's syndrome), autosomal-dominant, sex-linked, and sporadic forms. The degree of neutropenia varies from mild to severe, causing manifestations from occasional skin infections to repeated, severe, life-threatening infections.

Bone marrow examination reveals marked reduction in neutrophilic precursors at different levels. In many instances there is a marked reduction of the granulocytes at the intermediate and/or late stages of maturation (Figure 12–2). These changes are often associated with abnormal morphology including cytoplasmic vacuolization, decreased primary and secondary granules, and nuclear abnormalities. Similar bone marrow changes have been observed in drug-induced granulocytopenia.

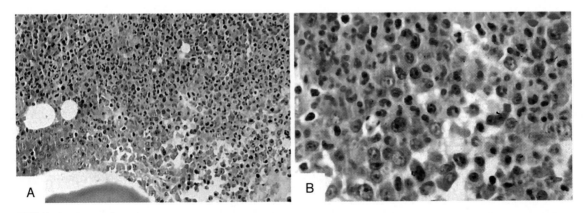

Figure 12–2. Agranulocytosis. Bone marrow biopsy section (*A*) and marrow smear (*B*) demonstrate marked erythroid preponderance and increased proportion of myeloblasts and promyelocytes. More mature myeloid elements are extremely rare.

LEUKEMOID REACTION

The term *leukemoid reaction* refers to extreme leukocytosis, particularly neutrophilia (Figures 12–3 and 12–4). Leukemoid reactions may simulate CML. The major features distinguishing leukemoid reaction from CML are:

Lack of or sparse early immature myeloid cells (myeloblasts, promyelocytes) in blood
Elevated leukocyte alkaline phosphatase (LAP) scores
Lack of basophilia
Presence of toxic granulation
Lack of Ph[1] chromosome (see Table 4–4, Chapter 4)

In some cases of leukemoid reaction, however, early myeloid cells including myeloblasts and promyelocytes may be present in the blood smears. Leukemoid reactions with absolute monocytosis of 1000/μL or greater may mimic chronic myelomonocytic leukemia (CMML).

Leukemoid reaction has been observed in a variety of conditions, such as acute and chronic bacterial infections, autoimmune disorders, burns, malignancies, hyperthyroidism, and Down syndrome. Cytokine therapy, such as treatment with granulocyte colony-stimulating factor (G-CSF) and granulocyte-macrophage colony-stimulating factor (GM-CSF), may also induce a leukemoid reaction (Figures 12–5 and 12–6).

Figure 12–3. Leukemoid reaction. Bone marrow biopsy sections (*A* and *B*) and marrow smears (*C* and *D*) demonstrate myeloid hyperplasia. The patient had pulmonary tuberculosis and marked peripheral blood leukocytosis.

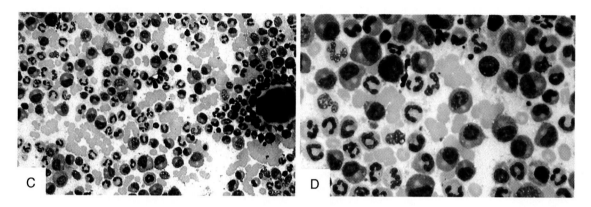

Figure 12–3. *Continued*

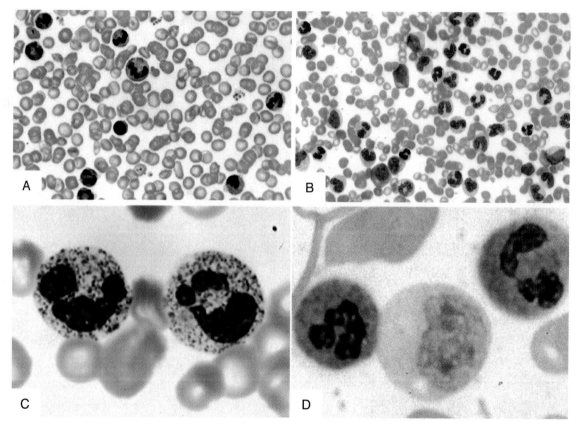

Figure 12–4. Leukemoid reaction. A relatively normal blood smear is presented for comparison (*A*). Blood smears of patients with leukemoid reactions demonstrate marked granulocytosis with moderate left shift (*B*). Toxic granulation is a frequent feature (*C*). There is also increased neutrophilic alkaline phosphatase activity (elevated leukocyte alkaline phosphatase [LAP] scores) (*D*).

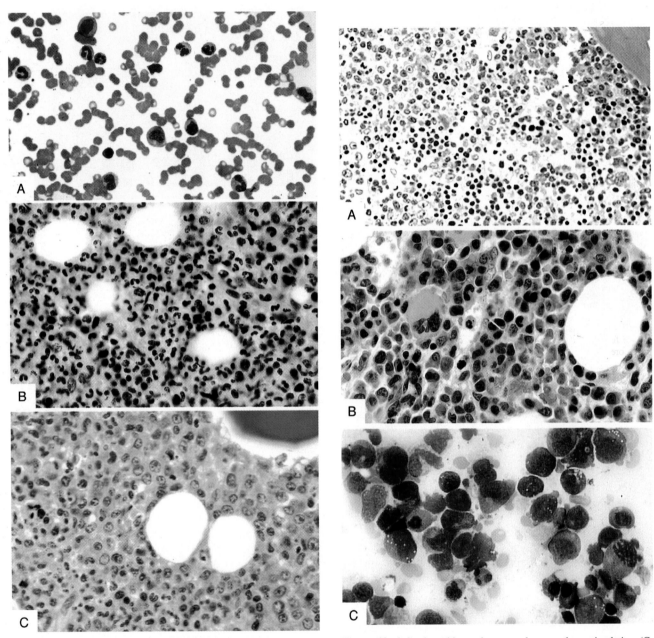

Figure 12–5. Leukemoid reaction, granulocyte-macrophage colony-stimulating factor (GM-CSF)-induced. *A*, Blood smear demonstrates granulocytosis with a shift to the left. Bone marrow clot (*B*) and biopsy (*C*) sections show a hypercellular marrow with marked myeloid preponderance.

Figure 12–6. Leukemoid reaction, granulocyte colony-stimulating (G-CSF)-induced. Bone marrow biopsy sections (*A* and *B*) demonstrate a hypercellular marrow with myeloid preponderance and left shift. Bone marrow smear (*C*) shows myeloid left shift with dysplastic changes.

EOSINOPHILIA

Eosinophilia is observed in a wide variety of conditions, such as protozoan and metazoan infections, allergic and inflammatory reactions, immunodeficiencies, autoimmune disorders, histiocytosis, malignancies, and hypereosinophilic syndrome (Figure 12–7).

Eosinophilia has been reported in a subtype of acute lymphoblastic leukemia (ALL) associated with t(5;14) and is a frequent finding in CML. A subtype of acute myelomonocytic leukeia (AML-M4) is associated with atypical eosinophilia and chromosomal aberrations of 16q22. Pa-

tients with a variety of solid tumors, such as bronchogenic carcinoma and medullary carcinoma of the thyroid gland, may also demonstrate eosinophilia.

Hypereosinophilic syndrome is a marked reactive eosinophilia of unknown etiology characterized by persistent eosinophilia equal to or greater than 1500/μL for 6 months or more. The eosinophils in hypereosinophilic syndrome are often atypical and may demonstrate abnormal nuclear segmentation and/or granulation. Bone marrow shows marked eosinophilia (usually >30%) with a shift to the left (see Figure 12–7).

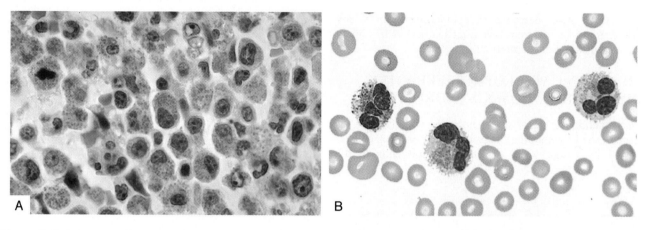

Figure 12–7. Hypereosinophilic syndrome. Bone marrow section (*A*) demonstrates marked eosinophilia with increased numbers of intermediate and mature forms, and blood smear (*B*) shows eosinophils with more than two nuclear segments. (From Naeim F: Pathology of Bone Marrow, 2nd ed. Baltimore, Williams & Wilkins, 1998, with permission.)

BASOPHILIA

Basophilia is observed in a wide variety of conditions, such as hypersensitivity reactions, autoimmune disorders,

ulcerative colitis, myeloproliferative disorders, and certain subclasses of acute myelogenous leukemia (AML) [AML-M3, AMLs with t(6;9)] (Figure 12–8).

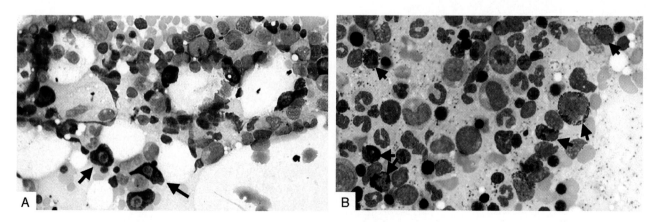

Figure 12–8. Mast cells and basophils. Bone marrow smear from a patient with myelodysplastic syndrome demonstrates increased mast cells (*A, arrows*). Bone marrow smear from a patient with chronic myelogenous leukemia shows increased numbers of basophils (*B, arrows*).

MASTOCYTOSIS

Bone marrow mastocytosis is observed in primary mast cell disorders as well as a variety of hematologic and nonhematologic conditions. Myeloproliferative disorders, lymphoproliferative disorders, MDS, AML, aplastic anemia, bone marrow fibrosis, chronic liver disease, and osteoporosis are conditions that may demonstrate increased bone marrow mast cells (see Figure 12–8).

Bone marrow involvement in mast cell disorders is usually focal or patchy with aggregate(s) of spindle-shaped mast cells against a fibrotic background. Mast cells contain purplish-black cytoplasmic granules. These granules are better demonstrated by Giemsa or toluidine blue stains. Also, detection of cytoplasmic tryptase (by cytochemical or immunoenzyme techniques) is helpful in the identification of the mast cells.

TRANSIENT MYELOPROLIFERATIVE DISORDER IN DOWN SYNDROME

This condition is observed in neonates with Down syndrome usually within the first month of birth. It is characterized by leukocytosis, presence of blast cells in the blood, and increased blast cells in the bone marrow (Figure 12–9). Blasts are predominantly of erythroid and/or megakaryocytic lineage. Cytogenetic studies, except for trisomy 21, are unremarkable. In most cases, the bone marrow and blood abnormalities disappear spontaneously after 4 to 6 weeks. This disorder, in a small proportion of the patients, evolves to AML.

Selected References

Barak Y, Nir E: Chédiak-Higashi syndrome. Am J Pediatr Hematol Oncol 9:42, 1987.

Horny HP, Ruck P, Kröber S, et al: Systemic mast cell disease (mastocytosis): General aspects and histopathological diagnosis. Histol Histopathol 12:1081, 1997.

Liang D-C, Ma S-W, Lu T-H, et al: Transient myeloproliferative disorder and acute myeloid leukemia: Study of six neonatal cases with long-term follow up. Leukemia 7:1521, 1993.

Malech HL, Nauseef WM: Primary inherited defects in neutrophil function: Etiology and treatment. Semin Hematol 34:279, 1997.

Marinone G, Roncoli B, Marinone MG Jr: Pure white cell aplasia. Semin Hematol 28:298, 1991.

Rothenberg ME: Eosinophilia. N Engl J Med 338:1592, 1998.

Shastri KA, Logue GL: Autoimmune neutropenia. Blood 81:1984, 1993.

Zipursky A, Brown EJ, Christensen H, et al: Transient myeloproliferative disorder (transient leukemia) and hematologic manifestations of Down syndrome. Clin Lab Med 19:157, 1999.

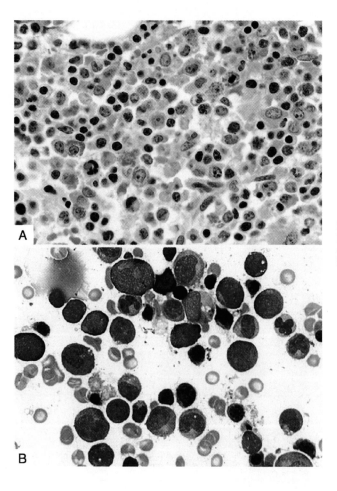

Figure 12–9. Transient myeloproliferative disorder in Down syndrome. Bone marrow biopsy section (*A*) and marrow smear (*B*) from a 3-week-old child with Down syndrome demonstrate marked myeloid left shift and increased blast cells.

CHAPTER 13

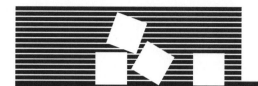

Lymphocytic Disorders

The nonneoplastic lymphoproliferative disorders, such as virus-associated reactive lymphocytosis, chronic polyclonal B-cell lymphocytosis, and benign bone marrow lymphoid aggregates, are briefly discussed in this chapter.

VIRUS-ASSOCIATED REACTIVE LYMPHOCYTOSIS

A wide variety of viruses, such as Epstein-Barr virus (EBV), cytomegalovirus (CMV), varicella-zoster virus, rubella virus, adenovirus, and the hepatitis viruses, may cause polyclonal reactive lymphocytosis. EBV infection is the classic example in this group, with a clinical manifestation known as infectious mononucleosis (IM).

EBV infects B lymphocytes and causes a polyclonal B-cell proliferation, which in turn initiates a polyclonal T-cell proliferation leading to suppression of the B cells. This self-limiting process is defective in X-linked lymphoproliferative syndrome, and the result is continuation of B-cell proliferation, and in some cases, development of malignant lymphoma.

Blood examination demonstrates lymphocytosis (usually $>4500/\mu L$) with a high proportion ($>20\%$) of activated (atypical) lymphocytes. The activated lymphocytes are large and polymorphic with abundant cytoplasm; round, oval, or irregular nucleus; and dense chromatin (Figures 13–1 and 13–2). The nucleoli are often small or inconspicuous. The cytoplasm demonstrates some degree of basophilia and may show scalloping of the cytoplasmic membrane around erythrocytes (see Figure 13–1). The lymphocytes are a mixture of B and T cells, often with a preponderance of suppressor/cytotoxic ($CD8^+$) cells. Bone marrow examination may reveal lymphocytosis with the presence of large pleomorphic atypical cells (see Figure 13–2). Small granulomas may also be present. IM is one of the major causes of infection-associated hemophagocytosis.

Clinical Aspects

The clinical symptoms include malaise, sweating, sore throat, headache, and fever, which are often associated with lymphadenopathy, splenomegaly, and hepatomegaly. EBV infection during infancy or childhood generally does not result in distinctive clinical symptoms, whereas approximately 50% of the infected individuals between ages 16 and 22 develop clinical symptoms.

Differential Diagnosis

Differential diagnosis includes malignant lymphoma and acute lymphoblastic leukemia (ALL). IM may simulate both Hodgkin's and non-Hodgkin's lymphomas, particularly in the affected lymph nodes. Some of the atypical lymphocytes may show binucleation and appear as Reed-Sternberg (RS) cells. However, the lesions usually lack nodal architectural effacement and the background polymorphic inflammatory infiltrate characteristics of Hodgkin's lymphoma. The atypical cells may also mimic neoplastic cells in large cell lymphomas, but they are polyclonal and consist of a mixture of activated B and T cells with no evidence of monotypic population.

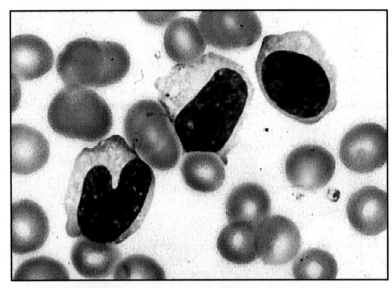

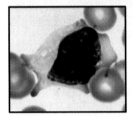
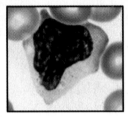
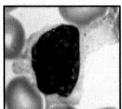

Figure 13–1. Virus-associated reactive lymphocytosis. Blood smears from patients with infectious mononucleosis demonstrate atypical (activated) lymphocytes. The lymphocytes are large and polymorphic with abundant cytoplasm; round, oval, or irregular nucleus; and dense chromatin. The nucleoli are often small or inconspicuous. The cytoplasm demonstrates some degree of basophilia and may show scalloping of the cytoplasmic membrane around erythrocytes.

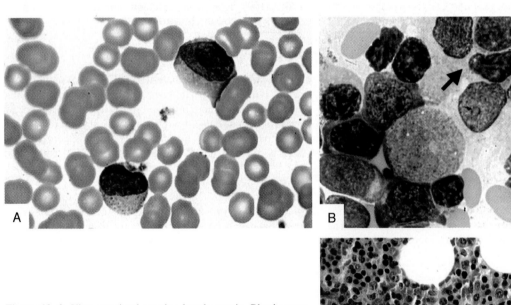

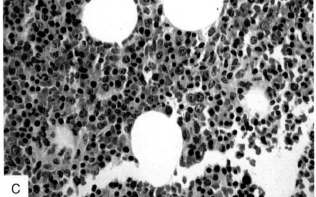

Figure 13–2. Virus-associated reactive lymphocytosis. Blood smear demonstrates two activated lymphocytes (A). They are polymorphic with abundant cytoplasm, variable nuclear shape, and dense nuclear chromatin; one shows cytoplasmic azurophilic granules. Bone marrow smear shows scattered atypical lymphocytes (B, arrow), but no lymphoid aggregate is noted in the biopsy section (C).

CHRONIC POLYCLONAL B-CELL LYMPHOCYTOSIS

Chronic or persistent polyclonal B-cell lymphocytosis is a rare condition. Most reported cases are in young to middle-aged women with a history of heavy smoking. There is also an association between this disorder and HLA-DR7. The blood lymphocyte count is elevated (ranging from 4000/μL to 20,000/μL), with the presence of activated as well as binucleated forms (Figures 13–3 and 13–4). Lymphocytes are polyclonal and positive for CD19, CD20, and CD22. They may express CD11c and CD25 but are usually negative for CD5. Bone marrow is unremarkable.

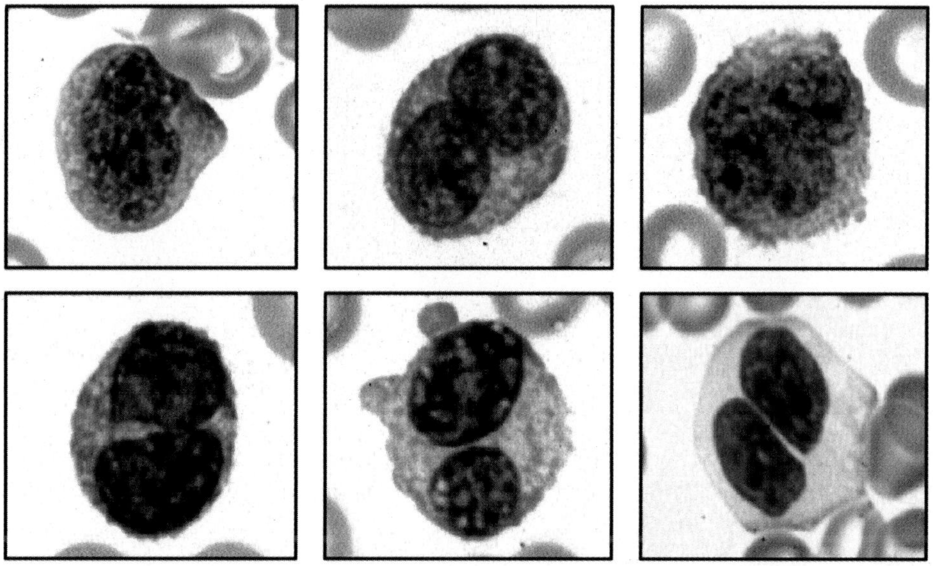

Figure 13–3. Chronic polyclonal B-cell lymphocytosis. Blood smears demonstrate nuclear irregularity, binucleation, and nuclear lobulation of the lymphocytes. These cells are polyclonal and, unlike CLL cells, which are usually CD5-positive, rarely express CD5.

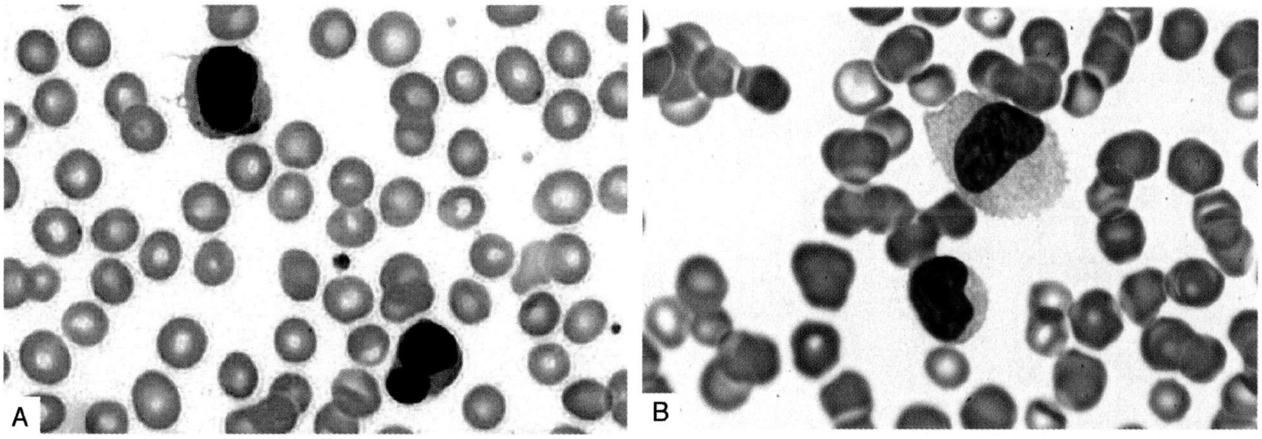

Figure 13–4. Chronic polyclonal B-cell lymphocytosis. Blood smears (*A* and *B*) demonstrate atypical lymphocytes with irregular nuclei and show variation in size and amount of cytoplasm.

BENIGN LYMPHOID AGGREGATES

Benign lymphoid aggregates are relatively common in the bone marrow sections. They are more frequent in women and older people. They consist of small, well-defined aggregates of mature lymphocytes, surrounded by fat or hematopoietic cells (Figures 13–5 to 13–9). Germinal centers are infrequent and are found in about 5% of the lymphoid aggregates (see Figures 13–7 and 13–8). Their presence suggests a reaction to a severe or chronic immunologic stimulation. Lymphoid aggregates are sometimes mixed with variable numbers of plasma cells, eosinophils, mast cells, and histiocytes/dendritic cells (reactive polymorphous lymphohistiocytic lesions). The polymorphous lesions may be large, poorly defined, or paratrabecular (see Figure 13–9).

Clinical Aspects

Lymphoid aggregates have been observed in association with autoimmune disorders, postsplenectomy status, drug reactions, viral infections (e.g., human immunodeficiency virus [HIV]), aplastic anemia, myeloproliferative disorders, myelodysplastic syndromes, and hematologic malignancies.

Differential Diagnosis

Differential diagnosis includes low-grade lymphomas such as small lymphocytic lymphoma/chronic lymphocytic leukemia, small cleaved and marginal zone lymphomas, and mantle cell lymphoma. The benign lymphoid aggregates are often well circumscribed, usually are not paratrabecular, and show no cellular atypia or evidence of monoclonality. The polymorphous lesions may mimic Hodgkin's or T-cell lymphomas.

Other Conditions Associated With Abnormal Lymphocyte Morphology

In addition to virus-associated atypical lymphocytosis and chronic polyclonal lymphocytosis, abnormal lymphocyte morphology has been observed in a variety of disorders, such as Chédiak-Higashi syndrome (large reddish-purple cytoplasmic granules), mucopolysaccharidosis (Alder-Reilly anomaly), and the juvenile type of neuronal ceroid-lipofuscinosis (cytoplasmic vacuolization) (Figure 13–10).

Selected References

Brown KA: Nonmalignant disorders of lymphocytes. Clin Lab 10:329, 1997.

Carr R, Fishlock K, Matutes E: Persistent polyclonal B-cell lymphocytosis in identical twins. Br J Haematol 96:272, 1997.

Farhi DC: Germinal centers in the bone marrow. Hematol Pathol 3:133, 1989.

Gordon DS, Jones BM, Browning SW, et al: Persistent polyclonal lymphocytosis of B lymphocytes. N Engl J Med 307:232, 1982.

Maeda K, Hyun BH, Rebuck MD: Lymphoid follicles in bone marrow aspirates. Am J Clin Pathol 67:41, 1977.

Maia DM, Garwacki CP: X-linked lymphoproliferative disease: Pathology and diagnosis. Pediatr Devel Pathol 2:72, 1999.

Mitterer M, Pescosta N, Fend F, et al: Chronic active Epstein-Barr virus disease in a case of persistent polyclonal B-cell lymphocytosis. Br J Haematol 90:526, 1995.

Navone R, Valpreda M, Pich A: Lymphoid nodules and nodular lymphoid hyperplasia in bone marrow biopsies. Acta Haematol 74:19, 1985.

Peter J, Ray CG: Infectious mononucleosis. Pediat Rev 19:276, 1998.

Pettet JD, Pease G, Cooper T: An evaluation of paraffin sections of aspirated marrow in malignant lymphomas. Blood 10:820, 1955.

Rywlin AM, Ortega RS, Dominguez CJ: Lymphoid nodules of bone marrow: Normal and abnormal. Blood 43:389, 1974.

Seemayer TA, Grierson H, Pirruccello SJ, et al: X-linked lymphoproliferative disease. Am J Dis Child 147:1242, 1993.

Straus SE, Cohen JI, Tosato G, et al: Epstein-Barr virus infections: Biology, pathogenesis, and management. Ann Intern Med 118:45, 1992.

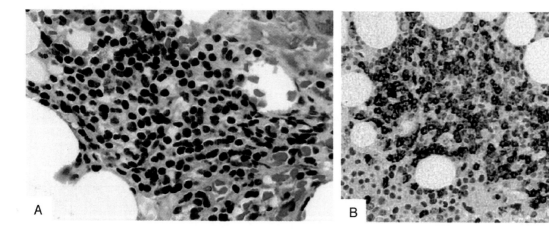

Figure 13–5. Benign lymphoid aggregate. Bone marrow biopsy section demonstrates a small lymphoid aggregate consisting of small, mature lymphocytes (*A*). Immunoperoxidase stains show a mixture of CD20-positive (*B*) and CD3-positive (*C*) cells.

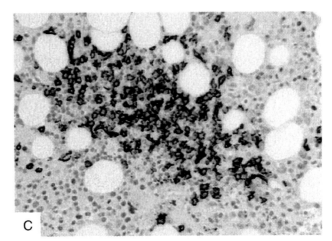

Figure 13–5 *Continued*

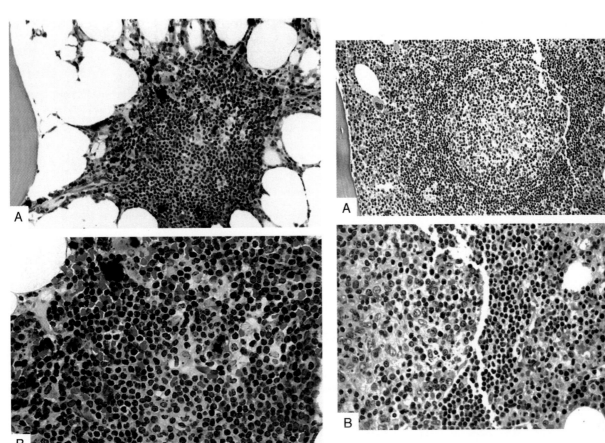

Figure 13–6. Benign lymphoid aggregate. Bone marrow biopsy section demonstrates a well-defined small lymphoid aggregate consisting of small, mature lymphocytes with scanty cytoplasm and round or slightly irregular nuclei (low-power [*A*] and high-power [*B*] views).

Figure 13–7. Benign lymphoid aggregate. Bone marrow biopsy section demonstrates a well-defined lymphoid aggregate with germinal center (low-power [*A*] and high-power [*B*] views).

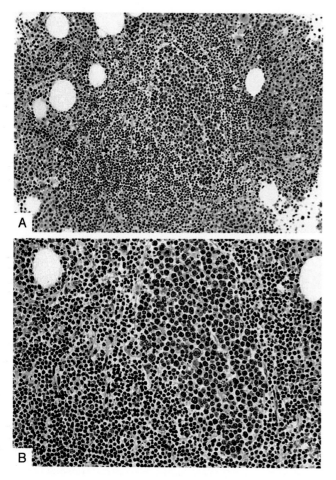

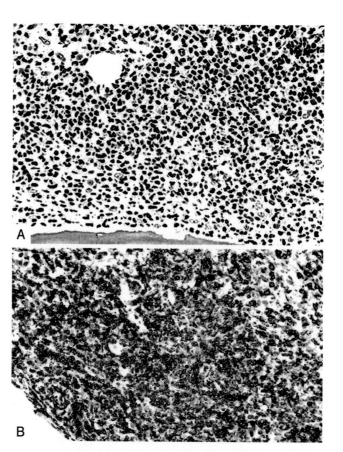

Figure 13–8. Benign lymphoid aggregate. Bone marrow biopsy section from a patient with chronic myelogenous leukemia demonstrates a lymphoid aggregate with germinal center (low-power [*A*] and high-power [*B*] views).

Figure 13–9. Atypical reactive lymphoid aggregate. Bone marrow biopsy section from a patient with a history of large B-cell lymphoma after completion of chemotherapy. *A,* There is an atypical paratrabecular lymphoid aggregate predominantly composed of mature, small- and medium-size lymphocytes with irregular nuclei. *B,* The immunoperoxidase stain shows sheets of CD3-positive cells. There was no evidence of CD20-positive cells and therefore no evidence of B-cell lymphoma (results not shown).

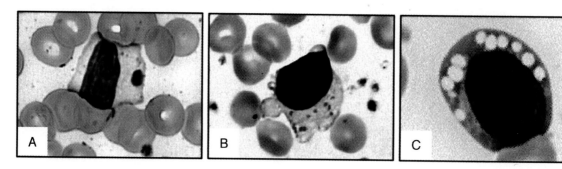

Figure 13–10. Abnormal lymphocytes. Blood smears demonstrate lymphocytes representing Chédiak-Higashi syndrome with a large reddish-purple cytoplasmic granule (*A*), a lymphocyte with Alder-Reilly anomaly (cytoplasmic azurophilic granules, *B*), and a lymphocyte with vacuolated cytoplasm found in the juvenile type of neuronal ceroid-lipofuscinosis (*C*).

CHAPTER 14

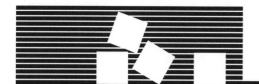

Anemias

Blood is the most informative sample for the diagnosis and classification of anemias. It provides valuable information regarding hemoglobin (Hb) and hematocrit (Hct) levels, red blood cell (RBC) indices, RBC morphology, reticulocyte count, serum iron, iron-binding capacity, ferritin, erythropoietin, folate, and vitamin B_{12} levels. It is the main resource for the evaluation of hemoglobinopathies. Bone marrow examination provides additional valuable information, such as the status of erythropoiesis, estimation of the stored iron, and presence or lack of marrow replacement by fibrosis, inflammatory process, or malignancy.

In general, anemias caused by RBC destruction or blood loss are characterized by reticulocytosis and bone marrow erythroid hyperplasia, whereas anemias due to bone marrow hypoplasia or ineffective erythropoiesis are associated with reticulocytopenia and a variable bone marrow cellularity ranging from profound hypocellularity to marked hypercellularity.

RED CELL APLASIA (HYPOPLASIA)

Red cell aplasia is divided into two types: acute and chronic. The acute red cell aplasia (aplastic crisis) has been associated with sickle cell anemia, hereditary spherocytosis, acquired hemolytic anemias, or other hemolytic disorders. The crisis is usually preceded by a bacterial or viral infection, and parvovirus appears to be the leading pathogen (Figure 14–1). The aplastic crisis is often transient and disappears by the termination of the infection.

Chronic red cell aplasia is of two types: congenital and acquired. The congenital red cell aplasia (Diamond-Blackfan anemia) is the result of a defect in the erythroid-committed stem cells, which are insensitive to erythropoietin and other growth-promoting factors. The disease develops in early childhood, usually before age 1. The acquired red cell aplasia often affects adults and has been associated with thymoma, autoimmune disorders, and lymphoid malignancies.

Bone marrow specimens show a reduction in the erythroid precursors, ranging from a virtual lack of erythroid elements (aplasia) to erythroid hypoplasia with the presence of early precursors and paucity of more mature forms (Figures 14–2 and 14–3; see Figure 14–1). Megaloblastic and dysplastic changes are often present. Myeloid and megakaryocytic lineages are unremarkable, or sometimes hyperplastic. Blood samples show absolute reticulocytopenia with elevated levels of the serum erythropoietin.

Differential Diagnosis

A decline in reticulocyte count with a sudden drop in the blood Hb level in a patient with hemolytic anemia strongly suggests aplastic crisis. Red cell aplasia is differentiated from hypoplastic forms of myelodysplastic syndrome by: (1) evidence of significant reduction in the erythroid series and (2) the presence of normal or near-normal myelopoiesis and megakaryocytopoiesis.

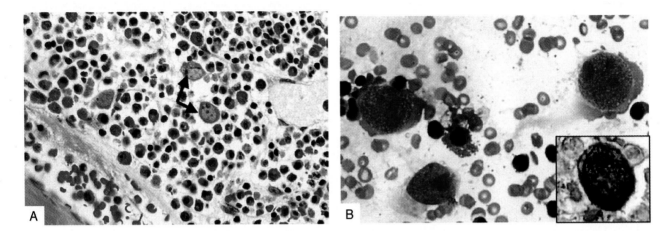

Figure 14–1. Erythroid aplasia. Bone marrow biopsy section (*A*) and marrow smear (*B*) of a patient with a history of autoimmune hemolytic anemia and recent parvovirus infection (aplastic crisis). Erythroid precursors are markedly reduced and only scattered giant erythroblasts are identified. The inset is a giant erythroblast stained for hemoglobin A (immunoperoxidase stain).

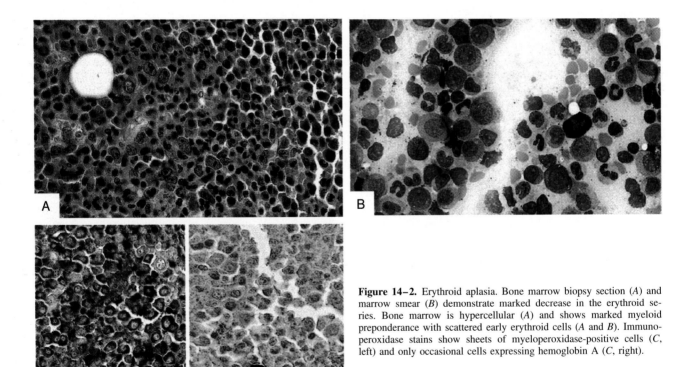

Figure 14–2. Erythroid aplasia. Bone marrow biopsy section (*A*) and marrow smear (*B*) demonstrate marked decrease in the erythroid series. Bone marrow is hypercellular (*A*) and shows marked myeloid preponderance with scattered early erythroid cells (*A* and *B*). Immunoperoxidase stains show sheets of myeloperoxidase-positive cells (*C*, left) and only occasional cells expressing hemoglobin A (*C*, right).

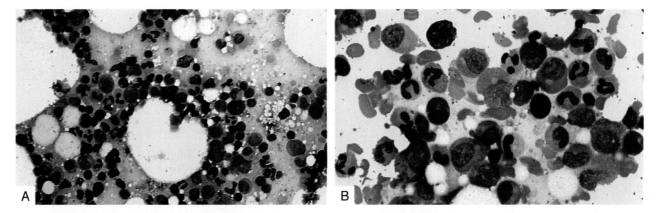

Figure 14–3. Erythroid aplasia. Bone marrow smear demonstrating marked decrease in the erythroid series in a patient with Diamond-Blackfan anemia (low-power [A] and high-power [B] views).

CONGENITAL DYSERYTHROPOIETIC ANEMIAS

Congenital dyserythropoietic anemias (CDA) are hereditary anemias characterized by dysplastic and ineffective erythropoiesis. Three major types are reported: type I (autosomal recessive), type II (autosomal recessive, positive for acidified serum test, and the most frequent type), and type III (autosomal dominant).

Bone marrow samples are hypercellular with marked erythroid preponderance. A high proportion of the erythroid precursors show bi- or multilobated nuclei, and many are binucleated (Figures 14–4 to 14–7). Nuclei in some of the binucleated cells may show chromatin bridging (see Figure 14–4). Megaloblastic changes and nuclear fragmentation are frequent findings. Abnormal morphologic changes are mostly observed in the middle and late stages of erythroid maturation. Pseudo-Gaucher cells and hemophagocytic histiocytes are sometimes present (see Figure 14–7). Very large multinucleated erythroid precursors (gigantoblasts) are observed in type III CDA (see Figure 14–7).

Blood smears demonstrate anisocytosis and poikilocytosis. Reticulocyte count is normal or slightly elevated.

Clinical Aspects

The age of onset varies from infancy to late adulthood. Anemia ranges from mild with no clinical symptoms to severe with hepatomegaly, jaundice, and gallstone formation.

Differential Diagnosis

Differential diagnosis includes megaloblastic anemia and myelodysplastic syndromes (MDS). In megaloblastic anemia, serum levels of folate or vitamin B_{12} are low and megaloblastic changes are also present in the myeloid series. The dysplastic changes are greater in CDA than MDS and, unlike CDA, MDS are often associated with multilineage bone marrow dysplasia. Also, neither MDS nor megaloblastic anemia are congenital disorders.

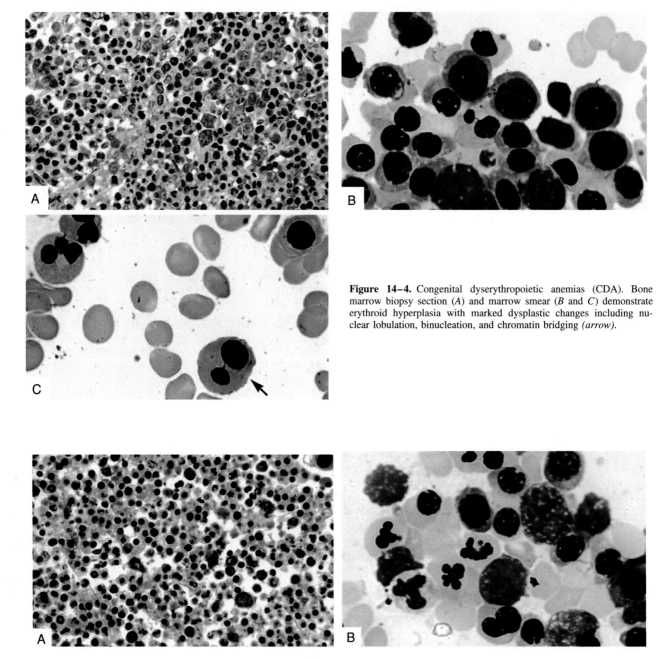

Figure 14–4. Congenital dyserythropoietic anemias (CDA). Bone marrow biopsy section (*A*) and marrow smear (*B* and *C*) demonstrate erythroid hyperplasia with marked dysplastic changes including nuclear lobulation, binucleation, and chromatin bridging *(arrow)*.

Figure 14–5. Congenital dyserythropoietic anemias (CDA). Bone marrow biopsy section (*A*) and marrow smear (*B*) demonstrate erythroid hyperplasia with dysplastic changes and marked nuclear lobulation.

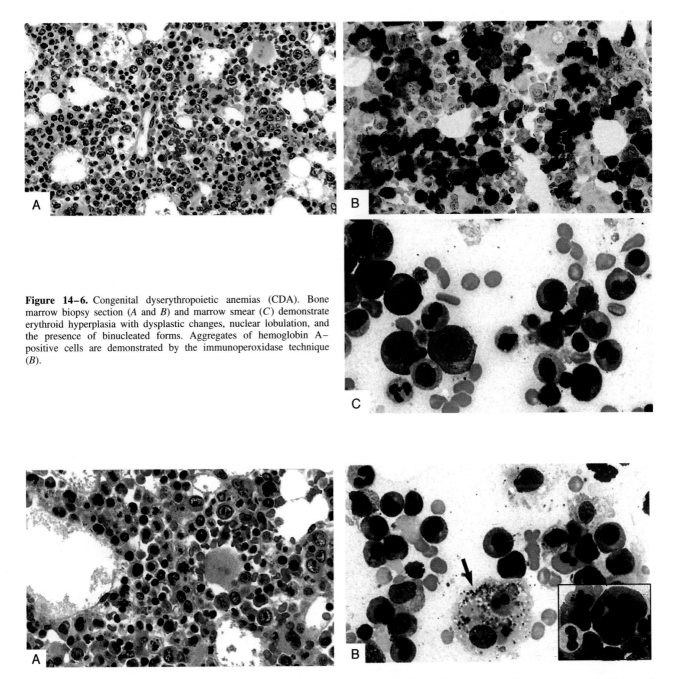

Figure 14–6. Congenital dyserythropoietic anemias (CDA). Bone marrow biopsy section (*A* and *B*) and marrow smear (*C*) demonstrate erythroid hyperplasia with dysplastic changes, nuclear lobulation, and the presence of binucleated forms. Aggregates of hemoglobin A–positive cells are demonstrated by the immunoperoxidase technique (*B*).

Figure 14–7. Congenital dyserythropoietic anemias (CDA). Bone marrow biopsy section (*A*) and marrow smear (*B*) demonstrate erythroid hyperplasia with dysplastic changes. A hemophagocytic histiocyte is present (*B, arrow*). The inset shows a giant multilobulated early erythroid cell.

MEGALOBLASTIC ANEMIAS

The basic defect in megaloblastic anemias is a delay in cell division due to a decline in the rate of DNA synthesis. The major etiologic factors are: (1) folic acid or vitamin B_{12} deficiencies and (2) congenital or acquired defects of purine or pyrimidin metabolism.

The impaired DNA synthesis delays cell division and leads to an ineffective erythropoiesis and premature destruction of the erythroid cells. The cytologic features are as follows (Figures 14–8 to 14–10):

The erythroid precursors are larger (megaloblastic) than their normal counterparts and show nuclear-cytoplasmic asynchrony. The cytoplasm is abundant and the nuclear chromatin is unevenly speckled. Final nuclear condensation (pyknosis) in late orthochromatic normoblasts is either delayed or fails to occur. Nuclear irregularity, lobulation, and/or fragmentation are frequent findings. The granulocytic series show dysplastic changes demonstrated by the presence of giant metamyelocytes and bands, and hypersegmented neutrophils (see Figures 14–9 and 14–10). There is also mild to moderate myeloid left shift. Megakaryocytes may show nuclear hypersegmentation. Megaloblastic changes are more striking in the intermediate and late stages of hematopoietic maturation.

Bone marrow sections and smears are hypercellular and demonstrate erythroid hyperplasia with a shift to the left (see Figures 14–8 to 14–10). Megaloblasts may appear in clusters as large immature cells with open chromatin and prominent nucleoli, resembling a leukemic process (see Figures 14–8 and 14–9).

Blood smears show anisopoikilocytosis with the presence of macro-ovalocytes (mean cell volume [MCV] often >115 fl) and reduced reticulocytes (see Figure 14–10). Hypersegmented neutrophils (six or more nuclear segments) are present. Basophilic stippling and Howell-Jolly bodies are frequently observed. Serum folate and vitamin B_{12} levels are low.

Clinical Aspects

Folic acid and vitamin B_{12} deficiencies are the most common causes of nutritional anemias after iron deficiency. Vitamin B_{12} deficiency, unlike folic acid deficiency, is associated with neurologic symptoms, resulting from degenerative changes in the dorsal and lateral columns of the spinal cord. A potentially fatal acute megaloblastic anemia has been reported in association with nitrous oxide anesthesia.

Differential Diagnosis

Megaloblastic changes are observed in MDS, erythroleukemia, and following chemotherapy. Also, patients treated with azidothymidine (AZT) for acquired immunodeficiency syndrome (AIDS) often show megaloblastic changes. In all these conditions serum folate and vitamin B_{12} levels are normal or elevated. Ringed sideroblasts or excess myeloblasts (>5%) may be present in various types of MDS, whereas they are absent in megaloblastic anemia. Coexistence of megaloblastic anemia and iron deficiency anemia may mask macrocytosis and megaloblastic changes, but usually giant metamyelocytes and bands and hypersegmented neutrophils are still present.

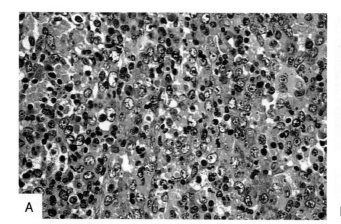
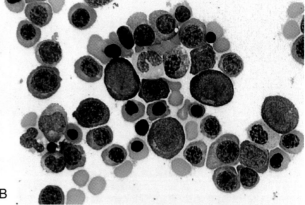

Figure 14–8. Megaloblastic anemia. Bone marrow biopsy section (*A*) demonstrates a hypercellular marrow with increased number of immature erythroid cells. Many of these cells show a large, round nucleus with finely dispersed chromatin and prominent nucleoli. Bone marrow smears (*B* and *C*) show megaloblastic changes with nuclear-cytoplasmic asynchrony. The cytoplasm is abundant and the nuclear chromatin is unevenly speckled. Nuclear irregularity, lobulation, and/or fragmentation are evident.

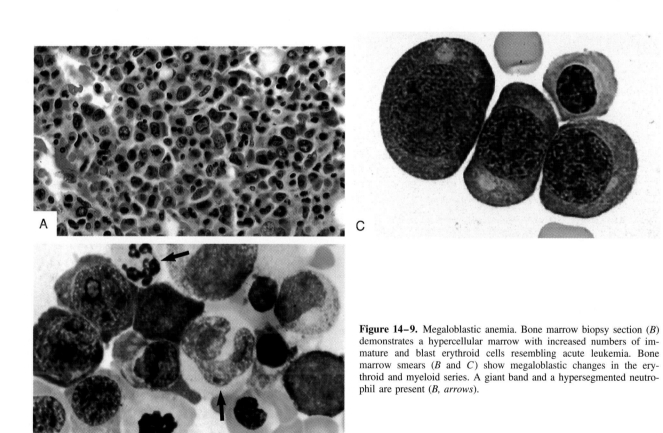

Figure 14–8 *Continued*

Figure 14–9. Megaloblastic anemia. Bone marrow biopsy section (*B*) demonstrates a hypercellular marrow with increased numbers of immature and blast erythroid cells resembling acute leukemia. Bone marrow smears (*B* and *C*) show megaloblastic changes in the erythroid and myeloid series. A giant band and a hypersegmented neutrophil are present (*B, arrows*).

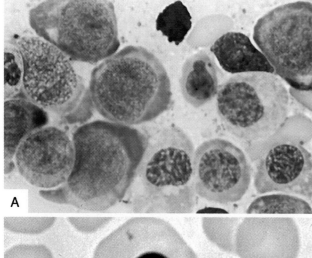

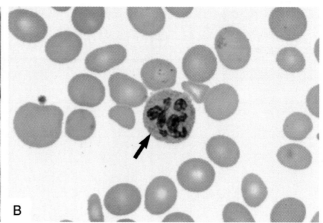

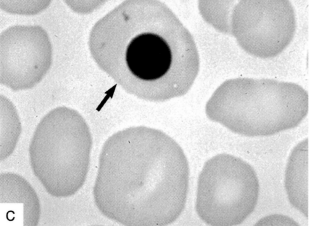

Figure 14–10. Megaloblastic anemia. Bone marrow smear (*A*) demonstrates megaloblastic erythroid cells. Blood smears show macro-ovalocytes (*B* and *C*). A hypersegmented neutrophil (*B, arrow*) and a nucleated red blood cell (RBC) with abundant cytoplasm (*C, arrow*) are present.

IRON DEFICIENCY ANEMIA

Iron deficiency is the most common cause of anemia, primarily affecting infants, women of reproductive age, and pregnant women. Inadequate dietary intake, blood loss, and iron malabsorption are the predominant etiologic factors.

Bone marrow sections are usually mildly to moderately hypercellular and often show erythroid preponderance and abundant megakaryocytes. Intermediate and late normoblasts are small and show scanty, ragged rims of poorly hemoglobinized cytoplasm. Lack of iron store is demonstrated by negative Prussian blue stain (Figure 14–11).

Blood smears show microcytic hypochromic RBCs (MCV < 80 fl) with various degrees of anisopoikilocytosis and ovalocytosis (see Figure 14–11). Target cells are present in severe cases. The reticulocyte count is low. Thrombocythemia is a frequent feature. Serum iron and ferritin levels are low, and total iron-binding capacity (TIBC) is elevated (Table 14–1).

Clinical Aspects

Many of the symptoms of anemia, such as fatigue, headache, and paresthesia, are often demonstrated before the complete depletion of iron store. Patients with chronic severe anemia may crave dirt, paint, or ice; demonstrate glossitis; and occasionally develop dysphagia associated with a postcricoid esophageal web (Plummer-Vinson syndrome).

Differential Diagnosis

Differential diagnosis includes thalassemia, anemia of chronic disease, and refractory anemia. In these conditions, bone marrow iron store is normal or increased and serum ferritin levels are elevated (see Table 14–1). Thalassemia shows an abnormal proportion of hemoglobin subtypes (see below).

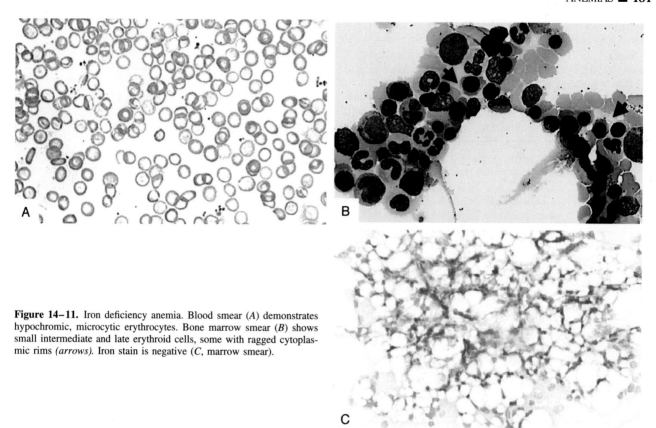

Figure 14–11. Iron deficiency anemia. Blood smear (*A*) demonstrates hypochromic, microcytic erythrocytes. Bone marrow smear (*B*) shows small intermediate and late erythroid cells, some with ragged cytoplasmic rims (*arrows*). Iron stain is negative (*C*, marrow smear).

Table 14–1

DIFFERENTIAL DIAGNOSIS OF IRON DEFICIENCY ANEMIA

	Serum			Bone Marrow	RBC
Anemia	*Fe*	*TIBC*	*Ferritin*	Iron Stain	Morphology
Iron deficiency	↓	↑	↓	Absent	Microcytic
Chronic disease	↑	↓	↑	↑	Micro- or normocytic
Refractory	↑	↑ or N	↑	↑, ringed sideroblasts	Micro- and/or macrocytic
Thalassemia	↑ or N	↑ or N	↑	↑	Microcytic

Fe = iron; TIBC = total iron-binding capacity; RBC = red blood cell; N = normal.

THALASSEMIAS

Thalassemias are a group of microcytic anemias caused by inherited defects in the production of one or more of the globin genes. There are two β genes (chromosomes 11) and four α genes (chromosomes 16). The defect results in an abnormal proportion of HbA ($\alpha2\beta2$), HbA2 ($\alpha2\delta2$), and HbF ($\alpha2\gamma2$). HbA, HbA2, and HbF consti-

tute over 95%, 3% or more, and less than 2% of the hemoglobin in normal individuals, respectively.

Thalassemias are divided into two major groups, β-thalassemia and α-thalassemia, based on the decrease or absence in production of β-chains or α-chains, respectively.

Beta-thalassemia consists of two types: (1) homozygous ($\beta-$thalassemia major) and (2) heterozygous

(β—thalassemia minor). **Alpha-thalassemia** consists of four different types: (1) silent carrier with three functional α genes; (2) α-thalassemia trait with two functional α genes; (3) HbH disease with one functional α gene; and (4) Bart's hydrops with no functional α gene.

Beta-thalassemia minor and α-thalassemia trait are associated with microcytosis, mild anemia, and no significant bone marrow changes. Beta-thalassemia major and HbH disease show severe microcytic anemia with the presence of the target cells, anisopoikilocytosis, basophilic stippling, Pappenheimer granules, and nucleated RBCs in the blood (Figures 14–12 and 14–13), and evidence of erythroid hyperplasia and increased iron stores in the bone marrow. The presence of HbH is demonstrated by the brilliant cresyl-blue stain, which displays greenish-blue inclusions in the affected RBCs (resembling golf balls). Hb Bart's is incompatible with extrauterine life.

Clinical Aspects

Thalassemias are prevalent in the Mediterranean basin, Middle East, Southeast Asia, and among African Americans. Clinical features vary from very mild, asymptomatic anemia to severe transfusion-dependent anemia.

Differential Diagnosis

Hereditary background distinguishes thalassemias from other microcytic anemias, such as iron deficiency or refractory anemias. In β—thalassemia, hemoglobin electrophoresis shows elevated proportions of HbA2 and HbF. The presence HbH is demonstrated by the brilliant cresyl-blue test.

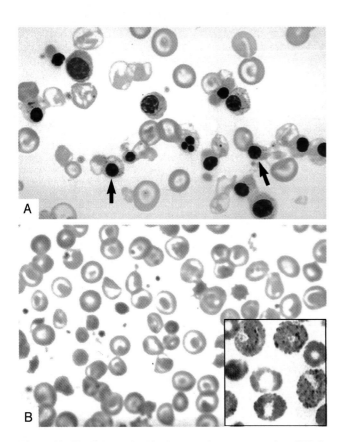

Figure 14–12. Thalassemia. Blood smears demonstrate nucleated RBCs (*A, arrow*) and numerous target cells (*A* and *B*). The inset shows HbH inclusions in α-thalassemia, creating a golfball appearance in the affected RBCs; brilliant cresyl-blue stain.

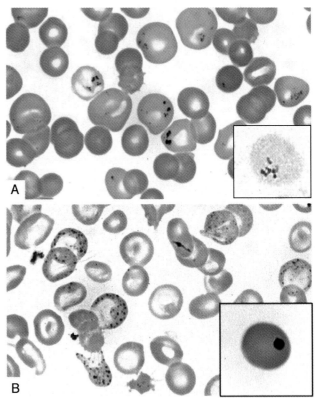

Figure 14–13. Thalassemia. Blood smears demonstrate erythrocytes with iron particles (Pappenheimer bodies) (*A*, Wright's stain and inset, iron stain), and basophilic stippling (*B*, Wright's stain). An erythrocyte with Howell-Jolly body is displayed in the inset (*B*).

SICKLE CELL ANEMIAS AND RELATED DISORDERS

Sickle cell anemias and related disorders are a group of hereditary hemoglobinopathies that are the result of mutations in the β-chain, or less frequently, α-chain of hemoglobin genes. The mutation results in the substitution of amino acids in globin chains leading to unstable hemoglobin molecules such as HbS, HbC, HbD, and HbE, or a combination of sickle-thalassemia disorders.

The extent of bone marrow cellularity and erythroid hyperplasia correlates with the severity of the anemia (Figure 14–14). Bone marrow expansion due to active erythropoiesis may lead to the reduction of bone mass and skeletal deformities.

Blood examination in severe cases shows anisopoikilocytosis with the presence of sickle cells, target cells, and nucleated RBCs (Figure 14–15). Mild to moderate leukocytosis and left shift are often present. In HbC disease, the abnormal hemoglobin may precipitate as rod-like crystals (see Figure 14–15).

Clinical Aspects

Sickle cell anemia (homozygous) is the most severe form of anemia in this group. Other forms, such as sickle cell trait (heterozygous), HbSC, HbC, HbD, HbE, HbS-β-thalassemia, and HbC-β-thalassemia, cause either no clinical symptoms or mild anemia. The heterozygous frequency of sickle cell disease is about 20% in Africans and about 8% in African Americans. Also, there is a high prevalence of sickle cell anemia in countries where malaria is epidemic.

The clinical symptoms of sickle cell anemia are manifested in the affected infants 8 to 10 weeks after birth. Affected children demonstrate growth retardation and skeletal abnormalities. Cerebrovascular ischemic events, papillary necrosis of the kidney, ischemic leg ulcers, recurrent infections, and repeated episodes of acute ischemic bone marrow suppression (sickle cell crisis) are among the complications.

Differential Diagnosis

Diagnosis of sickle cell anemia is based on the family history and demonstration of HbS crystals on routine blood smears, sickle cell preparations, and/or by hemoglobin electrophoresis. Bone marrow samples during sickle cell crisis may demonstrate marked hypocellularity, resembling aplastic anemia.

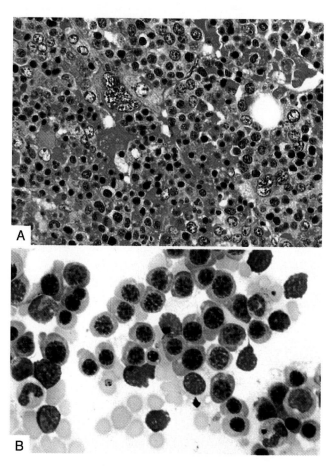

Figure 14–14. Erythroid hyperplasia is a frequent finding in patients with hemolytic anemia. Bone marrow biopsy section (*A*) and marrow smear (*B*) demonstrate large aggregates of erythroid precursors consistent with erythroid hyperplasia.

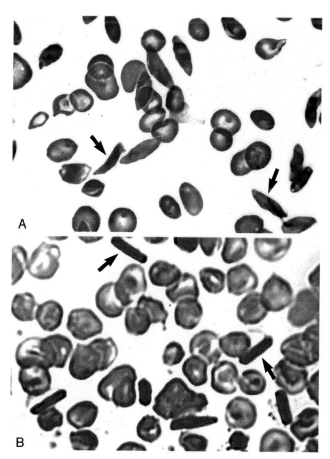

Figure 14–15. Hemoglobin S and C disorders. Blood smears demonstrate sickle cells (*A, arrows*) and hemoglobin C crystals (*B, arrows*).

RED BLOOD CELL MEMBRANE SKELETON DEFECTS

A group of hemolytic anemias are caused by defects of RBC membrane skeleton and are characterized by abnormal shape of the RBCs. Spherocytosis, elliptocytosis, acanthocytosis, and stomatocytosis are included in this group.

Hereditary spherocytosis is the most common type in this group and is caused by a defect in β-spectrin (autosomal dominant) or α-spectrin (autosomal recessive) synthesis. Blood examination reveals spherocytes (Figure 14–16), elevated RBC osmotic fragility, and, often, some degree of reticulocytosis. Anemia may range from mild to severe. Splenomegaly is common.

Hereditary spherocytosis is distinguished from other spherocytic anemias, such as autoimmune hemolytic anemia, by a negative Coombs' test and from unstable hemoglobins by the lack of Heinz bodies.

Hereditary elliptocytosis consists of a diverse group of hemolytic anemias characterized by the presence of oval, elliptical, or elongated erythrocytes caused by deficiencies of spectrin, protein 4.1, or glycophorin C (Figure 14–17).

Acanthocytosis is a condition characterized by erythrocytes with multiple irregularly shaped and randomly distributed cytoplasmic projections. Acanthocytes (spur cells) are differentiated from echinocytes (burr cells), which show numerous short, evenly distributed cytoplasmic projections (Figure 14–18).

Acanthocytosis is observed in a variety of conditions, such as severe liver disease, abetalipoproteinemia, cystic fibrosis, anorexia nervosa, and hypothyroidism.

Stomatocytosis is characterized by the presence of cup- or bowl-shaped erythrocytes, which in blood smears appear as cells with a wide transverse slit or stoma (see Figure 14–17). Stomatocytosis is either acquired or hereditary. The acquired form has been reported in alcoholism, hepatic diseases, cardiovascular disorders, and malignancies. The hereditary form in most instances is an autosomal dominant disorder associated with a defect in protein 7 synthesis.

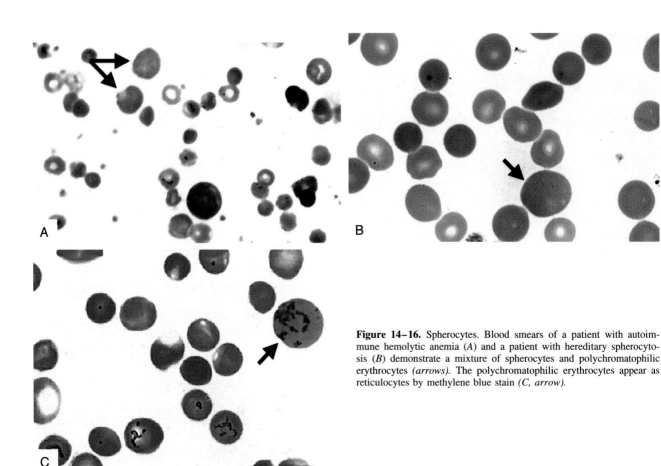

Figure 14–16. Spherocytes. Blood smears of a patient with autoimmune hemolytic anemia (*A*) and a patient with hereditary spherocytosis (*B*) demonstrate a mixture of spherocytes and polychromatophilic erythrocytes *(arrows)*. The polychromatophilic erythrocytes appear as reticulocytes by methylene blue stain *(C, arrow)*.

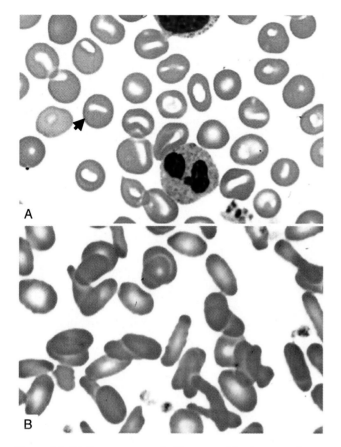

Figure 14–17. Stomatocytes and elliptocytes. Blood smears demonstrate stomatocytes *(A, arrow)* and elliptocytes *(B)*.

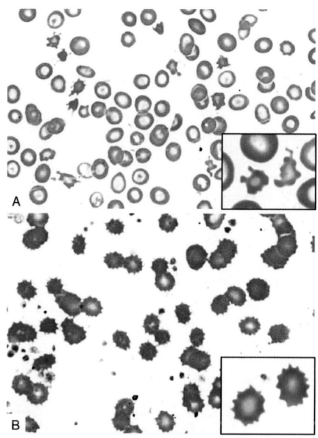

Figure 14–18. Acanthocytes and echinocytes. Blood smears demonstrate acanthocytes (spur cells) with uneven irregular cytoplasmic projections *(A)* and echinocytes (burr cells) with numerous, short, evenly distributed cytoplasmic projections *(B)*.

HEMOLYTIC ANEMIAS SECONDARY TO ERYTHROCYTE ENZYME DEFICIENCIES

Erythrocyte metabolic activities require numerous enzymes to maintain the functional and structural integrity of the RBCs, such as the adenosine triphosphatase (ATPase)-dependent cation pump. Red cell enzyme deficiencies may lead to a hemolytic anemia, which is usually normochromic and normocytic. The bone marrow response to the hemolytic process is erythroid hyperplasia. Glucose-6-phosphate dehydrogenase deficiency and pyruvate kinase deficiency are the two most prominent erythrocyte enzyme deficiencies.

AUTOIMMUNE HEMOLYTIC ANEMIA

Autoimmune hemolytic anemia (AIHA) is characterized by evidence of autoimmunity against erythrocytes, *in vivo* destruction of red cells, and bone marrow erythroid hyperplasia. The erythrocyte destruction is either intravascular or extravascular. Intravascular hemolysis is a complement-induced process within the vascular space, whereas in extravascular hemolysis, the antibody-coated red cells are removed by macrophages in tissues outside of the vascular space.

The autoantibodies are of two types: warm-reacting and cold-reacting.

The warm-reacting antibodies are of IgG type and lead to hemolysis by damaging the RBC membrane and creating RBC fragments and spherocytes. Blood smears show anisopoikilocytosis, spherocytosis, reticulocytosis, the presence of nucleated RBCs, and various degrees of granulocytosis and thrombocytosis (see Figure 14–16). In severe cases, there may be a leukoerythroblastic blood picture. Bone marrow demonstrates erythroid hyperplasia.

The cold-reacting antibodies are of IgM class and show enhanced activity below 37° C and particularly below 20°

C. In cold weather, with cooler peripheral circulation, the cold-reacting antibodies bind to the erythrocytes and mediate complement fixation, leading to RBC agglutination and hemolysis (Figure 14–19).

AIHA is distinguished from hereditary spherocytosis by lack of family history and positive Coombs' (antiglobulin) tests.

Patients with hemolytic anemia may develop parvovirus infection (Figure 14–20) leading to aplastic crisis and a sudden drop in the reticulocyte count.

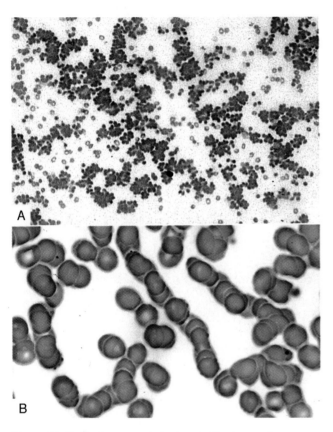

Figure 14–19. Erythrocyte agglutination. *A*, Blood smear demonstrates erythrocyte agglutination caused by the presence of cold-reacting IgM antibodies. *B*, Blood smear displays rouleaux formation for comparison.

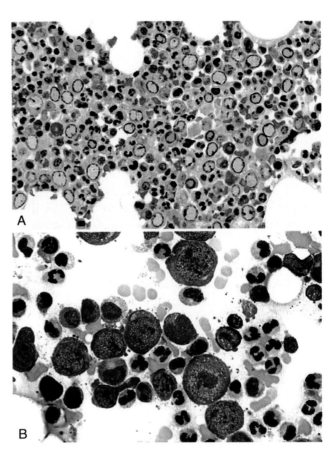

Figure 14–20. Parvovirus infection. Bone marrow section (*A*) demonstrates numerous erythroid precursors with nuclear viral inclusions. Bone marrow smear (*B*) shows several megaloblasts with coarse chromatin and nuclear inclusions. Intermediate and late erythroid precursors are rare (also, see Figure 14–1).

NONIMMUNE HEMOLYTIC ANEMIAS

Hemolysis may occur in a variety of nonimmune acquired conditions, such as trauma, heat, infection, and hypersplenism.

Traumatic injury to the RBCs has been observed in patients with aortic valve disease, disseminated intravascular coagulopathy (DIC), thrombotic thrombocytopenic purpura (TTP), generalized vasculitis, and carcinomatosis. It has also been reported after walking or running long distances, bongo drumming, and karate exercises. These conditions cause RBC fragmentation and hemolysis (Figure 14–21). Thermal damage is often associated with spherocytosis and RBC fragmentation (Figure 14–22). Certain microorganisms cause hemolysis by releasing membrane-damaging substances (such as phospholipases and hemolysins) or by invading and destroying the RBCs (such as malaria) (Figure 14–23). Also, macrophage activation in certain bacterial or viral infections is sometimes associated with extensive erythrophagocytosis and anemia (see Chapter 11).

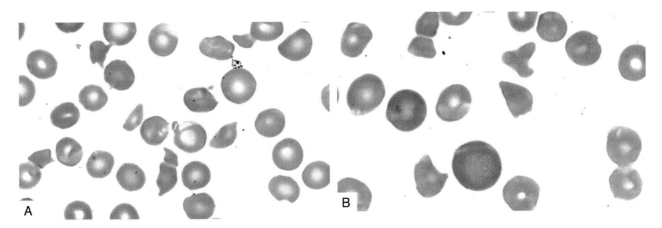

Figure 14–21. Schistocytes. Blood smears (*A* and *B*) demonstrate fragmented erythrocytes (schistocytes). Schistocytes have been observed in a wide variety of conditions, such as aortic valve disease, disseminated intravascular coagulopathy (DIC), thrombotic thrombocytopenic purpura (TTP), generalized vasculitis, and carcinomatosis.

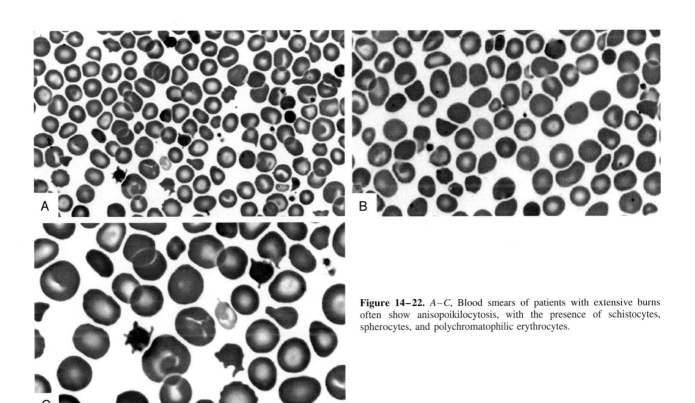

Figure 14–22. *A–C*, Blood smears of patients with extensive burns often show anisopoikilocytosis, with the presence of schistocytes, spherocytes, and polychromatophilic erythrocytes.

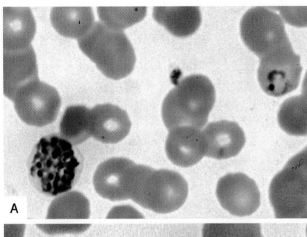

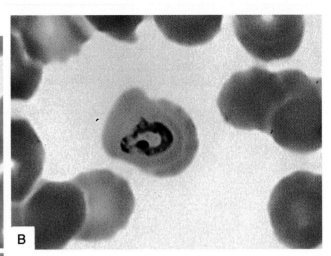

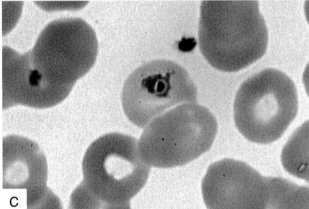

Figure 14–23. Malaria parasites. *A–C*, Blood smears demonstrate ring and schizont forms of malaria parasites in the erythrocytes.

OTHER TYPES OF ANEMIA

Anemia of Chronic Disease

Anemia associated with chronic disorders, such as chronic infections, chronic inflammations, and malignancies, is characterized by ineffective erythropoiesis, shortening of the RBC lifespan, low serum iron and iron-binding capacity, and increased bone marrow iron store (Figure 14–24). Bone marrow is normocellular or moderately hypocellular with no evidence of erythroid hyperplasia. Blood smears show normochromic/normocytic or hypochromic/microcytic RBCs.

Anemia of Chronic Renal Failure

Suppressive effects of uremia on erythropoiesis, plasma inhibitors of heme synthesis, and decreased erythropoietin production are among contributing factors in anemia of chronic renal failure. Anemia is usually normochromic/normocytic and bone marrow is normo- or hypocellular and may show paratrabecular fibrosis and erythroid hypoplasia (Figure 14–25).

Anemia of Endocrine Disorders

Some of the patients with endocrine disorders, such as pituitary, thyroid and adrenal gland insufficiencies, may develop anemia. Anemia is usually normochromic/normocytic and is associated with bone marrow erythroid hypoplasia.

Myelophthisic Anemia

Bone marrow–occupying lesions, such as hematopoietic malignancies, metastatic neoplasms, lipid storage diseases, and fibrosis, reduce normal hematopoiesis and cause anemia (Figure 14–26). Bone marrow metastasis and fibrosis are often associated with anisopoikilocytosis, and the presence of teardrop-shaped RBCs, nucleated RBCs, and immature granulocytic forms (leukoerythroblastic blood picture).

Selected References

Beutler E, Miwa S, Palek J: Hemolytic anemias. Rev Invest Clin Suppl: 162, 1994.

Bowie LJ, Reddy PL, Beck KR: Alpha thalassemia and its impact on other clinical conditions. Clin Lab Med 17:97, 1997.

Carmel R: Megaloblastic anemias. Curr Opin Hematol 1:107, 1994.

Delaunay J: Genetic disorders of the red cell membrane. Crit Rev Oncol Hematol 19:79, 1995.

Dessypris EN: The biology of pure red cell aplasia. Semin Hematol 28: 275, 1991.

Finch C: Regulators of iron balance in humans. Blood 84:1697, 1994.

Harris JW: Parvovirus B-19 for the hematologist. Am J Hematol 39: 119, 1992.

Higgs DR: β-thalassemia. Clin Haematol 6:57, 1993.

Lane PA: Sickle cell disease. Pediatr Clin North Am 43:639, 1996.

Lin CK, Lin JS, Chen SY, et al: Comparison of hemoglobin and red blood cell distribution width in the differential diagnosis of microcytic anemia. Arch Pathol Lab Med 116:1030, 1992.

Means RT, Jr: Pathogenesis of the anemia of chronic disease: A cytokine mediation anemia. Stem 13:32, 1995.

Olivieri NF: The beta-thalassemias. N Engl J Med 341:99, 1999.

Sackey K: Hemolytic anemia: Part 1. Ped Rev 20:152, 1999.

Smith LA: Autoimmune hemolytic anemias: Characteristics and classification. Lab Sci 12:110, 1999.

Tse WT, Lux SE: Red blood cell membrane disorders. Br J Haematol 104:2, 1999.

Weatherall DJ, Clegg JB: Thalassemia—a global public health problem. Nat Med 2:847, 1996.

Wickramasinghe SN, Illum N, Wimberley PD: Congenital dyserythropoietic anaemia with novel intra-erythroblastic and intra-erythrocytic inclusions. Br J Haematol 79:322, 1991.

Wright MS, Smith LA: Laboratory investigation of autoimmune hemolytic anemias. Clin Lab Sci 12:119, 1999.

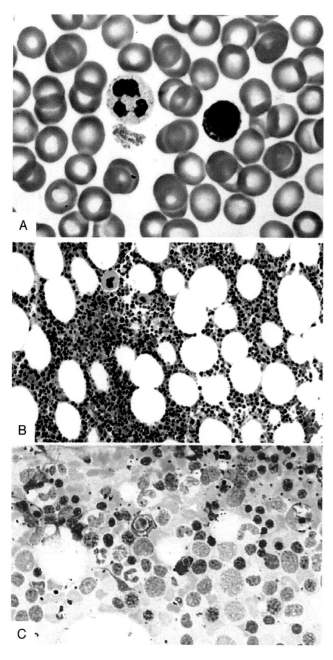

Figure 14–24. Anemia of chronic disease. *A,* Blood smear demonstrates normochromic and normocytic RBCs. Bone marrow clot section (*B*) displays a normocellular marrow, and iron stain shows abundant stored iron (*C,* marrow smear).

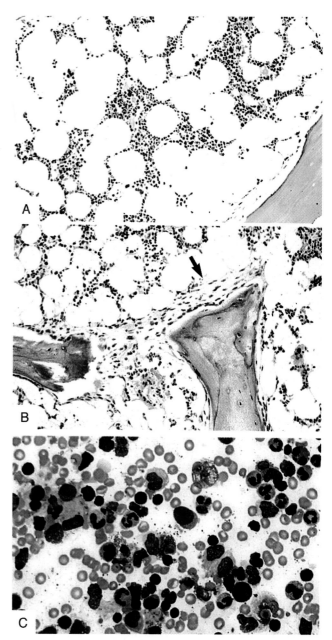

Figure 14–25. Anemia associated with chronic renal failure. Bone marrow biopsy sections demonstrate a hypocellular marrow with paratrabecular fibrosis (*A* and *B, arrow*). Bone marrow smear (*C*) shows reduced proportion of the erythroid precursors.

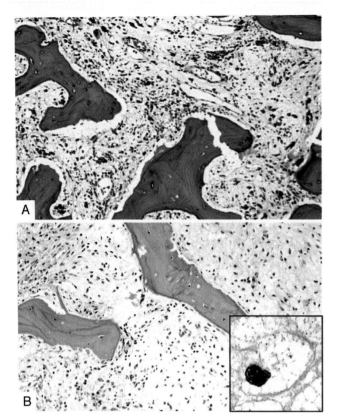

Figure 14–26. Myelophthisic anemia. Bone marrow-occupying lesions, such as fibrosis (*A*) or Niemann-Pick disease (*B*), reduce normal hematopoiesis and cause anemia (often pancytopenia).

CHAPTER 15

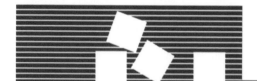

Disorders of the Megakaryocytic Lineage

Production of the platelets, similar to the other bone marrow activities, is a complex process. It involves proliferation and maturation of the committed colony-forming unit (CFU-M) cells, nuclear polyploidy and development of megakaryocytes, and finally, formation and release of the platelets.

Qualitative and quantitative abnormalities of megakaryocytes are often observed in clonal multipotent stem cell defects, such as myelodysplastic syndromes, myeloproliferative disorders, and leukemias (see Chapters 3, 4, and 5). Other disorders of megakaryocytes and platelets are briefly discussed in this chapter.

MEGAKARYOCYTIC HYPOPLASIA

Megakaryocytic hypoplasia or aplasia is one of the predominant features of congenital or acquired aplastic anemias. Lack or decreased production of megakaryocytes is rare without marrow aplasia and has been reported in a variety of viral infections, chronic alcoholism, and prolonged administration of prednisone, estrogen, and interferon. Thromboxytopenia–absent radius (TAR) syndrome is congenital megakaryocytic hypoplasia associated with thrombocytopenia, bilateral aplasia of the radii, and cardiac and/or renal malformations.

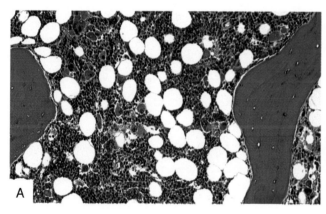

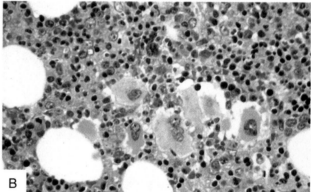

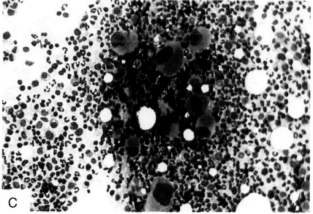

Figure 15–1. Megakaryocytosis and thrombocythemia. Bone marrow biopsy sections (*A* and *B*) and marrow smear (*C*) demonstrate increased megakaryocytes.

MEGAKARYOCYTOSIS AND THROMBOCYTOSIS

Reactive megakaryocytosis and thrombocytosis have been observed in iron deficiency anemia, acute infections, and bone marrow metastasis, as well as postsplenectomy. Clonal stem cell defects such as myeloproliferative disor-

ders, myelodysplastic syndromes, and acute megakaryoblastic leukemia (AML-M7) are often associated with megakaryocytosis and thrombocytosis. Unlike reactive megakaryocytosis and thrombocytosis, megakaryocytes and platelets in this group often demonstrate dysplastic changes (Figures 15–1 to 15–5).

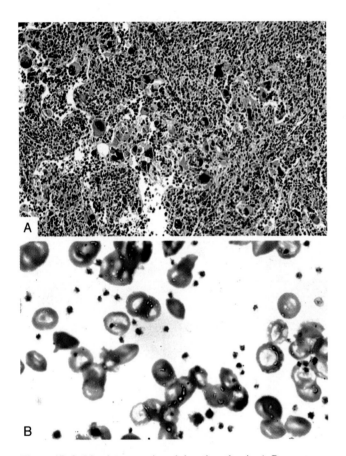

Figure 15–2. Megakaryocytosis and thrombocythemia. *A,* Bone marrow biopsy section from a patient with essential thrombocythemia demonstrates a hypercellular marrow with increased megakaryocytes. *B,* Blood smear shows thrombocythemia.

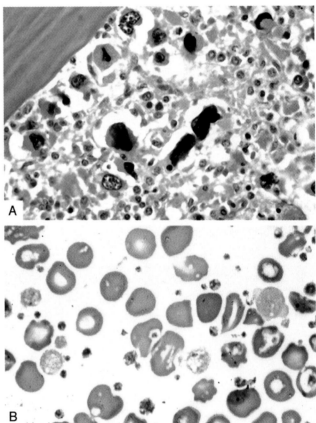

Figure 15–3. Megakaryocytosis and thrombocythemia. *A,* Bone marrow biopsy section from a patient with myelofibrosis with myeloid metaplasia demonstrates marked megakaryocytosis. *B,* Blood smear displays numerous giant platelets, some of which are hypogranular.

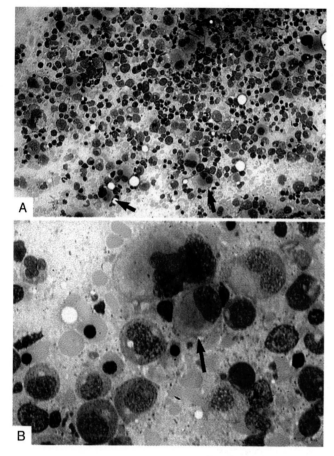

Figure 15–4. Megakaryocytosis. Bone marrow smears (*A* and *B*) from a patient with refractory anemia with excess blasts demonstrate numerous micromegakaryocytes (*arrows*).

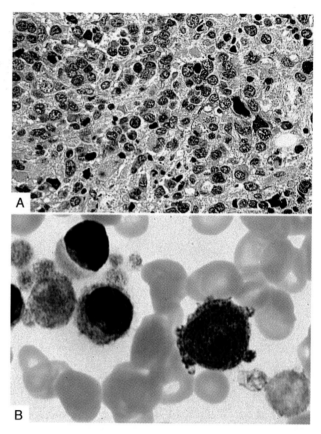

Figure 15–5. Megakaryoblasts. *A*, Bone marrow biopsy section from a patient with AML-M7 demonstrates clusters of blast cells. *B*, Blood smear shows blast cells with cytoplasmic budding and giant platelets. Immunophenotypic studies showed expression of CD42, CD61, and factor VIII by the blast cells, confirming their megakaryocytic origin (result not shown).

THROMBOCYTOPENIA

Impaired platelet production or increased platelet destruction leads to thrombocytopenia. Bone marrow hypoplasia, congenital deficiency of megakaryocytes, bone marrow replacement by fibrosis or neoplastic cells, drugs, radiation, certain infections, and malnutrition may cause reduction in megakaryocytes and consequently thrombocytopenia. Increased platelet destruction is often associated with megakaryocytosis and is caused by immunologic or nonimmunologic mechanisms. Autoimmune thrombocytopenic purpura and thrombotic thrombocytopenic purpura are selected as examples of thrombocytopenias and are briefly discussed in this chapter.

Autoimmune Thrombocytopenic Purpura

Autoimmune thrombocytopenic purpura (AITP) *(idiopathic thrombocytopenic purpura)* is an antibody-mediated disorder. Antibodies are usually raised against platelet membrane glycoproteins, such as GPIIb/IIIa, GPIb/IX, and GPV. Most of the antibodies are of the IgG class and can cross the placenta.

Bone marrow examination reveals an adequate or increased number of megakaryocytes. Megakaryocytes are pleomorphic, ranging from small mononuclear types to giant multilobulated forms (Figure 15–6). Some megakaryocytes may demonstrate less granular cytoplasm.

Blood examination reveals thrombocytopenia. Platelets vary in size and shape.

Clinical Aspects

There are two clinical forms of AITP: acute and chronic. Acute AITP is predominantly a childhood disease, affecting children between the ages of 2 and 9. Thrombocytopenia is severe and is often preceded by a viral infection. Spontaneous remission is observed in the majority of the patients within 6 to 12 months.

Chronic AITP is primarily observed in adults between the ages of 20 and 50 with a female:male ratio of about 3:1. Spontaneous remission is less frequent in the chronic form.

Differential Diagnosis

AITP is distinguished from impaired platelet production by the presence of adequate or increased numbers of megakaryocytes in the bone marrow. Other conditions associated with thrombocytopenia are myelodysplastic syndromes, leukemias, infections, drugs, and disseminated intravascular coagulation (DIC). Reduction in platelet count could be also caused by the ethylenediaminetetraacetic acid (EDTA)-dependent agglutinins (pseudothrombocytopenia).

Thrombotic Thrombocytopenic Purpura

The clinicopathological features of thrombotic thrombocytopenic purpura (TTP) are thrombocytopenia, microangiopathic hemolytic anemia, abnormal renal function, and neuropathy.

The most prominent pathologic process in TTP is the development of platelet/fibrin thrombi in capillaries and arterioles. The microthrombi are observed in various organs, such as the kidney, brain, adrenal gland, and heart. Microthrombi are rarely detected in bone marrow biopsy sections. Bone marrow is normocellular and demonstrates adequate or increased numbers of megakaryocytes.

Blood examination displays severe thrombocytopenia and anemia with anisopoikilocytosis, reticulocytosis, and the presence of fragmented and nucleated red blood cells (RBCs).

Clinical Aspects

The most frequent clinical manifestation is purpura, but epistaxis, hemoptysis, and other hemorrhagic episodes may also be present. The clinical course is either acute or chronic. The acute form has a grave outcome with a high rate of mortality. The chronic form is less frequent and has a better clinical outcome than the acute form.

Differential Diagnosis

Differential diagnosis includes conditions that are associated with hemolysis and thrombocytopenia, such as Evan's syndrome (autoimmune hemolytic anemia with thrombocytopenia), microangiopathic hemolytic anemias, DIC, and systemic lupus erythematous.

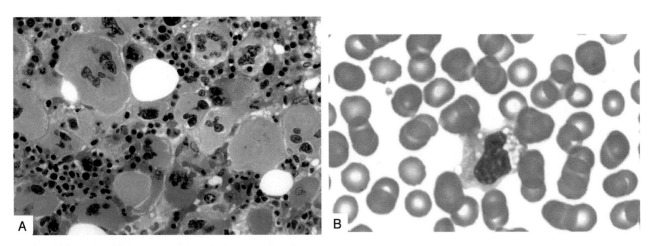

Figure 15–6. Immune-associated thrombocytopenic purpura. *A,* Bone marrow biopsy section demonstrates numerous megakaryocytes with several large forms. *B,* Blood smear displays a marked decrease in platelets.

QUALITATIVE PLATELET DISORDERS

Qualitative platelet disorders affect hemostasis by the change in platelet interactions with coagulation factors and/or blood vessels. These disorders are either congenital or acquired.

Congenital Platelet Disorders

Congenital platelet defects include disorders of the platelet adhesion or aggregation, deficiency of the platelet secretory granules, or disorders in the release of the platelet contents. Some of these disorders may show abnormal bone marrow and/or blood morphologic changes. For example, in Bernard-Soulier syndrome (platelet adhesion defect), blood platelet count is reduced and platelets are large, up to two to five times their normal size. However, bone marrow is unremarkable by light microscopic examination. In alpha-granule deficiency (gray platelet syndrome), the affected platelets are less granular than normal platelets and appear gray in blood smears stained with Wright's stain (Figure 15–7).

Acquired Platelet Disorders

Acquired platelet disorders are common and are found in association with consumption of a variety of foods, a large number of drugs, and many pathologic conditions, such as cardiopulmonary bypass, chronic renal disease, and hematologic disorders.

Abnormal platelet function and morphology has been observed in myelodysplastic syndromes, myeloproliferative disorders, and acute myelogenous leukemia. Morphologic changes include small and giant megakaryocytes with nuclear hypo- or hyperlobulation, and variation in platelet size and granulation.

Selected References

Chong BH: Diagnosis, treatment and pathophysiology of autoimmune thrombocytopenias. Crit Rev Oncol Hematol 20:271, 1995.

Eldor A: Thrombotic thrombocytopenic purpura: Diagnosis, pathogenesis and modern therapy. Bail Clin Haematol 11:475, 1998.

Gillis S: The thrombocytopenic purpuras: Recognition and management. Drugs 51:942, 1996.

Lages B, Sussman II, Levine SP, et al: Platelet alpha granule deficiency associated with decreased P-selectin and selective impairment of thrombin-induced activation in a new patient with gray platelet syndrome (alpha-storage pool deficiency). J Lab Clin Med 129:364, 1997.

López JA, Andrews RK, Afshar-Kharghan V, et al: Bernard-Soulier syndrome. Blood 91:4397, 1998.

Porta C, Caporali R, Montecucco C: Thrombotic thrombocytopenic purpura and autoimmunity: A tale of shadows and suspects. Haematologica 84:260, 1999.

Rand ML, Wright JF: Virus-associated idiopathic thrombocytopenic purpura. Transfusion Sci 19:253, 1998.

Sadowitz D, Souid AK, Terndrup TE: Idiopathic thrombocytopenic purpura in children: Recognition and management. Pediatr Emerg Care 12:222, 1996.

Westerman DA, Grigg AP: The diagnosis of idiopathic thrombocytopenic purpura in adults: Does bone marrow biopsy have a place? Med J Aust 170:216, 1999.

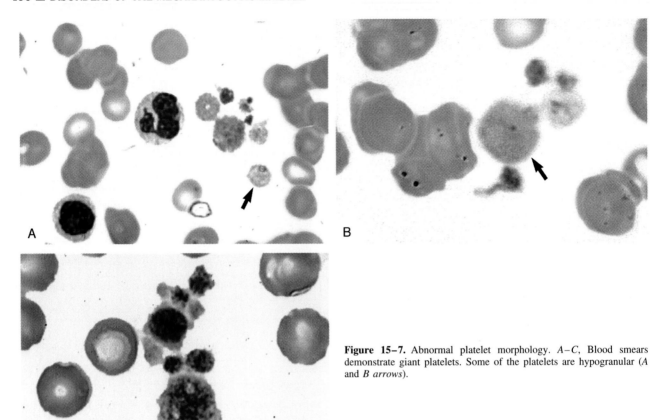

Figure 15–7. Abnormal platelet morphology. *A–C*, Blood smears demonstrate giant platelets. Some of the platelets are hypogranular (*A* and *B arrows*).

CHAPTER 16

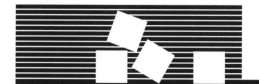

Bone Marrow Hypoplasia

Hypoplasia ("aplasia") of hematopoietic lineages is primarily due to inadequate quantity and/or functional defect of multipotent stem cells. Hypoplasia is associated with bone marrow hypocellularity and pancytopenia. Familial and acquired aplastic anemias, and paroxysmal nocturnal hemoglobinuria, are classic examples in this category and will be briefly discussed in this chapter.

FAMILIAL APLASTIC ANEMIAS

Familial or constitutional aplastic anemias are autosomal recessive disorders with a high prevalence in the South African population. A defect in the ability to repair DNA damage appears to play a major role in the pathogenesis of these disorders, and linkage studies suggest genetic abnormalities, defined by five complementation groups.

The bone marrow in the early stage of the disease is hyper- or normocellular, but eventually becomes markedly hypocellular (Figure 16–1). The biopsy sections show a fatty marrow with small foci of hematopoietic cells, which are predominantly of erythroid series. Bone mar-

row smears are hypocellular and consist predominantly of stromal cells. There is usually a high proportion of mast cells, plasma cells, lymphocytes, and macrophages. The morphologic features are similar to that of acquired aplastic anemia, and therefore are not pathognomonic.

Blood examination reveals pancytopenia. Anemia is usually normochromic/normocytic, but in some cases is macrocytic. The reticulocyte count is low.

Clinical Aspects

Familial aplastic anemia has two clinical manifestations: with physical abnormalities (Fanconi's anemia) and without physical abnormalities (Estren-Dameshek anemia). Physical abnormalities include growth retardation, patchy hyperpigmentation of skin (café au lait spots), renal hypoplasia, and skeletal abnormalities. Patients with Fanconi's anemia have a higher risk of developing myelodysplastic syndrome and acute myelogenous leukemia than the normal population.

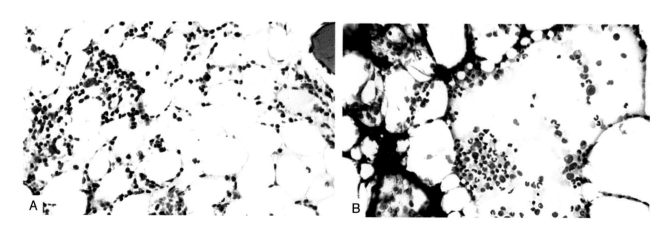

Figure 16–1. Bone marrow hypoplasia (Fanconi's anemia). Bone marrow biopsy section (*A*) and marrow smear (*B*) demonstrate a markedly hypocellular marrow with small aggregates of hematopoietic cells.

ACQUIRED APLASTIC ANEMIA

Acquired aplastic anemia is divided into *idiopathic* (with no known etiology) and *secondary* (with known etiology). A wide variety of factors have been reported as possible causes of secondary aplastic anemia, including drugs and chemicals, radiation, viral infections, and alteration in the immune system.

Bone marrow biopsy sections are the most valuable samples for the estimation of the extent of bone marrow hypoplasia (Figure 16–2). The bone marrow cellularity is often less than 25% of the normal range. Small foci of hematopoietic cells, predominantly erythroid, are present. Bone marrow smears are hypocellular and consist predominantly of stromal cells. Erythroid dysplasia and megaloblastic changes are sometimes present. Occasionally, the marrow smears may appear normocellular or even hypercellular. There is usually a high proportion of mast cells, plasma cells, lymphocytes, and macrophages.

Blood examination displays pancytopenia with reduced reticulocyte count. Anemia is usually normochromic and normocytic but may appear macrocytic in some cases. Neutrophils may show toxic granulation and an elevated leukocyte alkaline phosphatase (LAP) score.

Clinical Aspects

Severe aplastic anemias are usually idiopathic or are secondary to viral hepatitis. They are characterized by the following criteria: (1) bone marrow cellularity of less than 25% of the normal range and (2) pancytopenia with at least two of the following three features—neutropenia of less than 500/μL, platelets lower than 20,000/μL, and reticulocyte count less than 1%.

The prognosis for untreated aplastic anemia patients is poor, with 1-year survival rate of around 20%. Bone marrow transplantation, if possible, is an effective therapeutic approach. Other alternatives include immunosuppressive therapy and administration of hematopoietic growth factors.

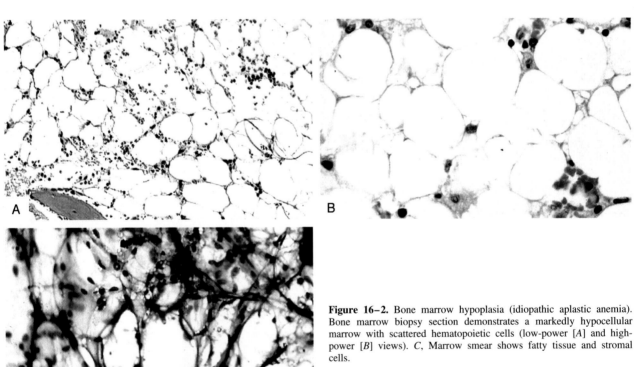

Figure 16–2. Bone marrow hypoplasia (idiopathic aplastic anemia). Bone marrow biopsy section demonstrates a markedly hypocellular marrow with scattered hematopoietic cells (low-power [*A*] and high-power [*B*] views). *C*, Marrow smear shows fatty tissue and stromal cells.

PAROXYSMAL NOCTURNAL HEMOGLOBINURIA

Paroxysmal nocturnal hemoglobinuria (PNH) is an acquired clonal disorder resulting in the decline or lack of the expression of surface membrane glycosylphosphatidyl-inositol (GPI)-linked proteins, such as CD14, CD16, CD24, CD48, CD55, CD58, CD59, CD67, and CD73 in the erythrocytes, leukocytes, and platelets. This membrane defect is associated with an increased sensitivity of the erythrocytes to complement-mediated lysis.

Bone marrow examination in most instances reveals a hypocellular marrow, with morphologic features similar to aplastic anemia (see Figure 16–2). However, unlike aplastic anemia, bone marrow iron store due to hemoglobinuria is reduced or absent. Some PNH cases may show a normo- or hypercellular marrow with myelodysplastic features.

Blood examination reveals a severe anemia with mild to moderate reticulocytosis. Anemia is normochromic and normocytic, and Ham's acid hemolysis test is positive. There is often granulocytopenia and thrombocytopenia, and the LAP score is low. The expression of GPI-linked proteins, such as CD55 and CD59, is reduced in erythrocytes and leukocytes.

Clinical Aspects

The peak incidence is between ages 25 and 35. The membrane defect in the majority of the PNH patients is permanent, leading to aplastic anemia and pancytopenia. PNH complications include iron deficiency (loss of hemosiderin and hemoglobin in the urine) and thrombosis (probably due to platelet activation by complement).

DIFFERENTIAL DIAGNOSIS

Bone marrow morphologic features in advanced congenital and acquired aplastic anemia and PNH are very similar and indistinguishable (see Figures 16–1 and 16–2). Additional clinicopathologic information is required for a more definitive diagnosis. Differential diagnosis also includes bone marrow hypoplasia secondary to chemotherapy and/or irradiation (Figure 16–3), as well as hypocellular variants of myelodysplastic syndrome, acute leukemia, and hairy cell leukemia (Figure 16–4). A summary of the differential diagnosis of aplastic anemia is presented in Table 16–1.

Selected References

Butturini A, Gale RP, Verlander PV, et al: Hematologic abnormalities in Fanconi anemia: An International Fanconi Anemia Registry Study. Blood 84:1650, 1994.

Carreau M, Buchwald M: Fanconi's anemia: What have we learned from the genes so far? Mol Med Today, May 4:201, 1998.

Dessypris EN: Aplastic anemia and pure red cell aplasia. Curr Opin Hematol 1:157, 1994.

Dokal I: Severe aplastic anemia including Fanconi's anemia and dyskeratosis congenita. Curr Opin Hematol 3:453, 1996.

Gordon-Smith EC, Rutherford TR: Fanconi anemia: Constitutional aplastic anemia. Semin Hematol 28:104, 1991.

Joenje H, Lo Ten Foe JR, Oostra AB, et al: Classification of Fanconi anemia patients by complementation analysis: Evidence for a fifth genetic subtype. Blood 86:2156, 1995.

Kwong YL, Lee CP, Chan TK, et al: Flow cytometric measurement of glycosylphosphatidyl-inositol-linked surface proteins on blood cells of patients with paroxysmal nocturnal hemoglobinuria. Am J Clin Pathol 102:30, 1994.

Tooze JA, Marsh JC, Gordon-Smith EC: Clonal evolution of aplastic anaemia to myelodysplasia/acute myeloid leukaemia and paroxysmal nocturnal haemoglobinuria. Leuk Lymphoma 33:231, 1999.

Young NS: Acquired aplastic anemia. JAMA 282:271, 1999.

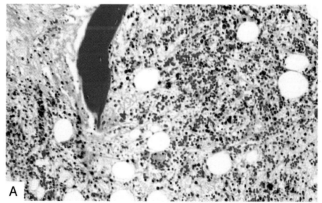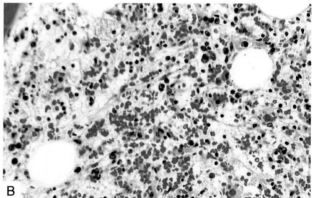

Figure 16–3. Postchemotherapy marrow. Bone marrow biopsy section from a patient with AML following chemotherapy demonstrates marked reduction in hematopoietic cells and increased proportion of stromal cells (low-power [A] and high-power [B] views).

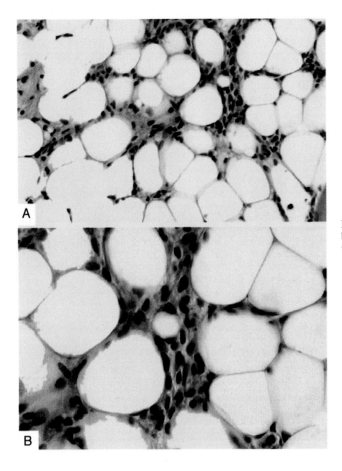

Figure 16–4. Hypocellular variant of hairy cell leukemia. Bone marrow biopsy sections (*A* and *B*) demonstrate a markedly hypocellular marrow with an interstitial lymphoid infiltrate.

Table 16–1
DIFFERENTIAL DIAGNOSIS OF APLASTIC ANEMIA (AA)

Disorder	Bone Marrow	Other Features
Congenital AA (Fanconi's)	Variable cellularity; often hypocellular	Chromosomal breakage; sometimes −7
Acquired AA	Hypocellular	Strong association with HLA-DR2 and -DRW3, in some reports
PNH	Variable cellularity; mostly hypocellular; reduced iron store	Positive Ham's test; reduced expression of the GPI-linked proteins; reticulocytosis
Hypocellular MDS	Dysplastic changes; often excess blasts (≥5%)	Abnormal cytogenetics, such as 5q-, -7, 8+
Hypocellular acute leukemia	Increases blasts (often >30%)	Abnormal cytogenetics
Hypocellular HCL	HCL cells; often fibrosis	TRAP+, expression of CD11c, CD22, CD25, and CD103

Adapted from Naeim F: Pathology of Bone Marrow, 2nd ed. Baltimore, Williams & Wilkins, 1998.
PNH = Paroxysmal nocturnal hemoglobinuria; HCL = Hairy cell leukemia; TRAP = Tartrate resistant acid phosphatase; GPI = glycosylphosphatidyl-inositol; MDS = myelodysplastic syndromes.

CHAPTER 17

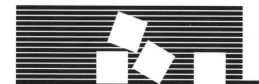

Bone Marrow Transplantation

Bone marrow transplantation is an attempt to restore blood cell formation in patients with defective hematopoiesis or those who receive myeloablative high-dose radiation and/or chemotherapy for neoplastic disorders. The source for the hematopoietic stem cells for transplantation is the patient (autologous transplant), the patient's identical twin (syngeneic transplant), or another human leukocyte antigen (HLA)-matched donor (allogeneic transplant). Stem cells are harvested from the donor's bone marrow or peripheral blood.

POST-TRANSPLANT BONE MARROWS

Bone marrow samples obtained a week following transplantation are markedly hypocellular and reveal occasional hematopoietic precursors. Samples obtained 1 to 3 weeks after transplantation often show evidence of bone marrow engraftment (Figures 17–1 and 17–2). The engrafted marrow demonstrates small clusters of erythroid and myeloid cells and occasional megakaryocytes. The myeloid clusters are often located around or close to the bone trabeculae, or tend to spread around the fatty tissue. In contrast, the erythroid cells usually appear as small, solid clusters in the middle of marrow space away from the bone trabeculae (see Figures 17–1 and 17–2). Dysplastic and megaloblastic changes are frequent findings. There are also various degrees of erythroid and myeloid left shift (Figure 17–3).

Bone marrow cellularity gradually increases by time, and large aggregates of hematopoietic cells composed of mixed-lineage hematopoietic precursors are formed (Figure 17–4). Also, dysplastic changes and left shift gradually disappear. Normocellularity is usually achieved within 8 to 12 weeks following transplantation.

During post-transplant bone marrow regeneration, an increase in proportion of hematogones (B-cell precursors) is noted. As mentioned before (see Chapter 1), these cells express TdT, CD10, CD19, HLA-DR, and sometimes CD34, and may mimic residual or relapsed leukemia, particularly in transplant recipients with a history of acute lymphoblastic leukemia (ALL) (see Figure 17–3).

Myeloid left shift and dysplasia and the presence of increased numbers of hematogones may create difficulties in distinguishing marrow engraftment/regeneration from residual/relapse acute myeloid or lymphoid leukemias. Cytogenetic and molecular studies, as well as additional follow-up bone marrow samplings will eventually help to separate these two processes.

Bone Marrow Graft Failure and Rejection

A small proportion of bone marrow recipients may show no morphologic, cytogenetic, or molecular evidence of engraftment. Also, the engrafted marrow in a proportion of the bone marrow recipients is rejected. During graft rejection, bone marrow cellularity declines and additional nonspecific changes, such as fat necrosis and increase in the number of plasma cells, lymphocytes, and/or histiocytes, are often noted. None of these changes are specific for graft rejection. Graft rejection is distinguished from lack of engraftment by evidence of marrow engraftment (by morphology, cytogenetic studies, or molecular techniques) prior to the graft failure.

Selected References

Armitage JO: Bone marrow transplantation. New Engl J Med 330:827, 1994.

Dernan NA, Bartsch G, Ash RC, et al: Analysis of 462 transplantations from unrelated donors facilitated by the National Marrow Donor Program. New Engl J Med 328:593, 1993.

Henon PR: Peripheral blood stem cell transplantation: Past, present and future. Stem Cells 11:154, 1993.

Mangan KF: Peripheral blood stem cell transplantation: From laboratory to clinical practice. Semin Oncol 22:202, 1995.

Naeim F: Pathology of Bone Marrow. Baltimore, Williams & Wilkins, 1997, p 453.

Naeim F, Smith G, Gale RP: Morphologic aspects of bone marrow transplantation in patients with aplastic anemia. Hum Pathol 35:61, 1977.

Passweg JR, Socie G, Hinterberger W, et al: Bone marrow transplantation for severe aplastic anemia: Has outcome improved? Blood 90: 858, 1997.

Rowlings, PA, Gale RP, Horowitz MM, Bortin MM: Bone marrow transplantation in leukemia. J Hematotherapy 3:235–243, 1994.

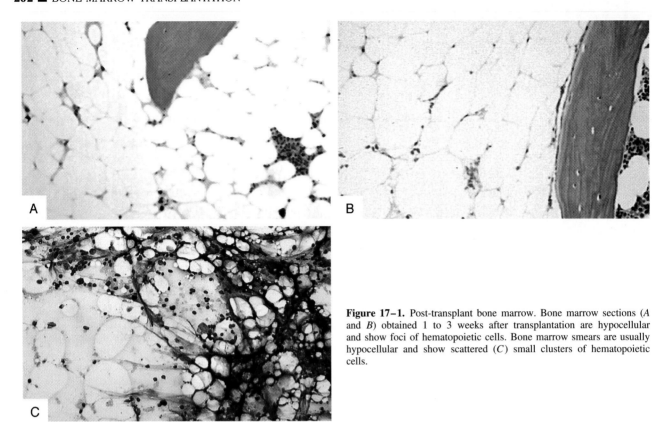

Figure 17–1. Post-transplant bone marrow. Bone marrow sections (*A* and *B*) obtained 1 to 3 weeks after transplantation are hypocellular and show foci of hematopoietic cells. Bone marrow smears are usually hypocellular and show scattered (*C*) small clusters of hematopoietic cells.

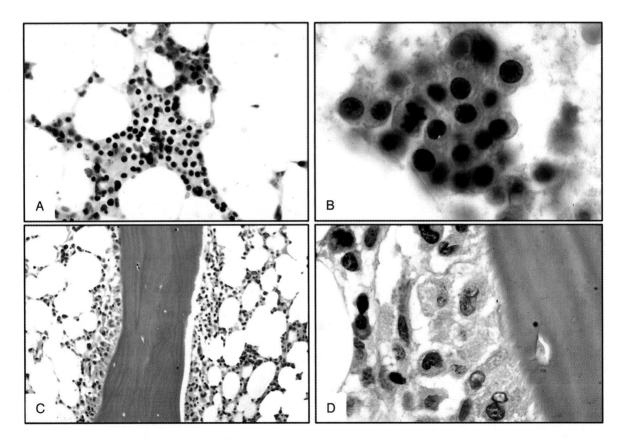

Figure 17–2. Post-transplant bone marrow. Bone marrow samples obtained 1 to 3 weeks after transplantation are hypocellular and show foci of hematopoietic cells. Erythroid clusters are usually far from the bone trabeculae (*A* and *B*) and myeloid clusters and are often close to bone trabeculae (*C* and *D*).

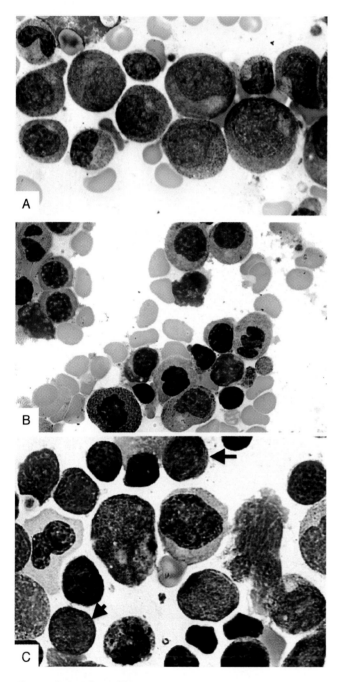

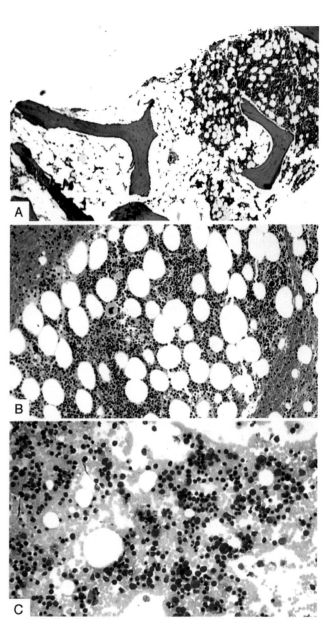

Figure 17–3. Post-transplant bone marrow. Bone marrow smears obtained 1 to 4 weeks after transplantation often show myeloid and erythroid left shift with dysplastic changes (*A* and *B*). Usually, there is also evidence of increased hematogones *(C, arrows)*.

Figure 17–4. Post-transplant bone marrow. Bone marrow samples obtained 4 to 8 weeks after transplantation show increased cellularity, which at early stages may appear patchy (*A*, biopsy section). The bone marrow cells are distributed more evenly at the later stages (*B*, clot section, and *C*, smear).

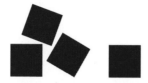

INDEX

Note: Page numbers in *italics* refer to illustrations; page numbers followed by t refer to tables.